complete cookery

# Healthy
# Meals

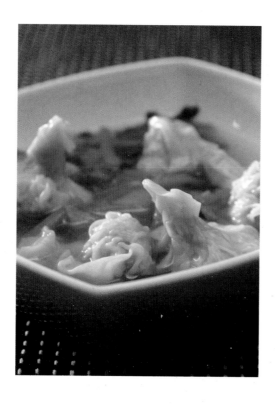

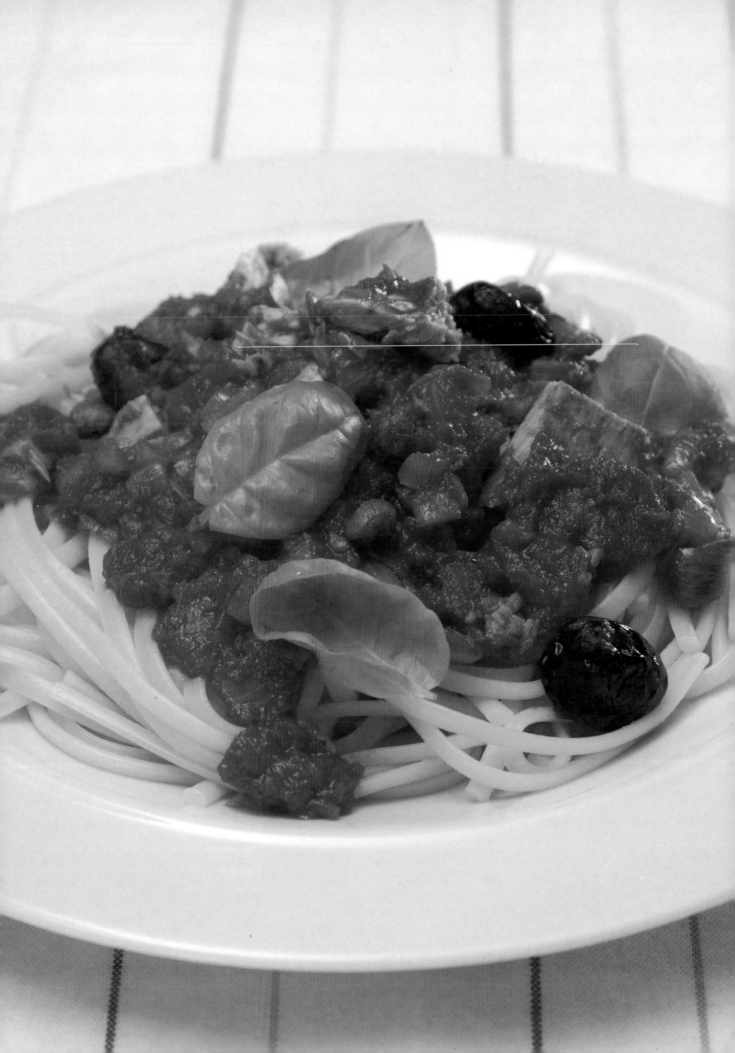

complete cookery

# Healthy
# Meals

Vicki Smallwood

Published by SILVERDALE BOOKS
An imprint of Bookmart Ltd
Registered number 2372865
Trading as Bookmart Ltd
Blaby Road
Wigston
Leicester LE18 4SE

© 2006 D&S Books Ltd

D&S Books Ltd
Kerswell,
Parkham Ash, Bideford
Devon, England
EX39 5PR

e-mail us at:- enquiries@d-sbooks.co.uk

ISBN   10 - 1-84509-441-7
       13 - 9-781-84509-441-6

DS0146. Complete Cookery: Healthy Meals

Creative Director: Sarah King
Project Editor: Claire Bone
Designer: Debbie Fisher
Photographer: Colin Bowling/Paul Forrester

Fonts: New York, Helvetica and Bradley Hand

Material from this book previously appeared 100 great recipes: Healthy Meals.

Printed in Thailand

1 3 5 7 9 10 8 6 4 2

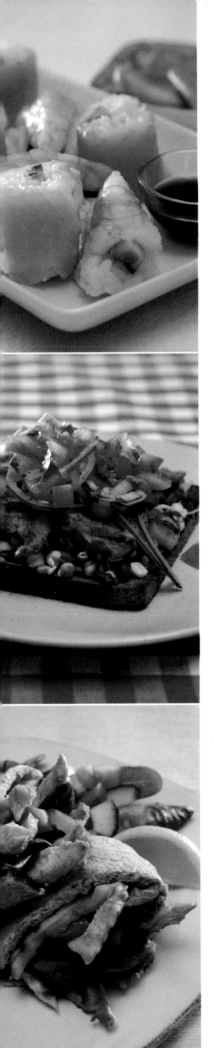

# Contents

# introduction

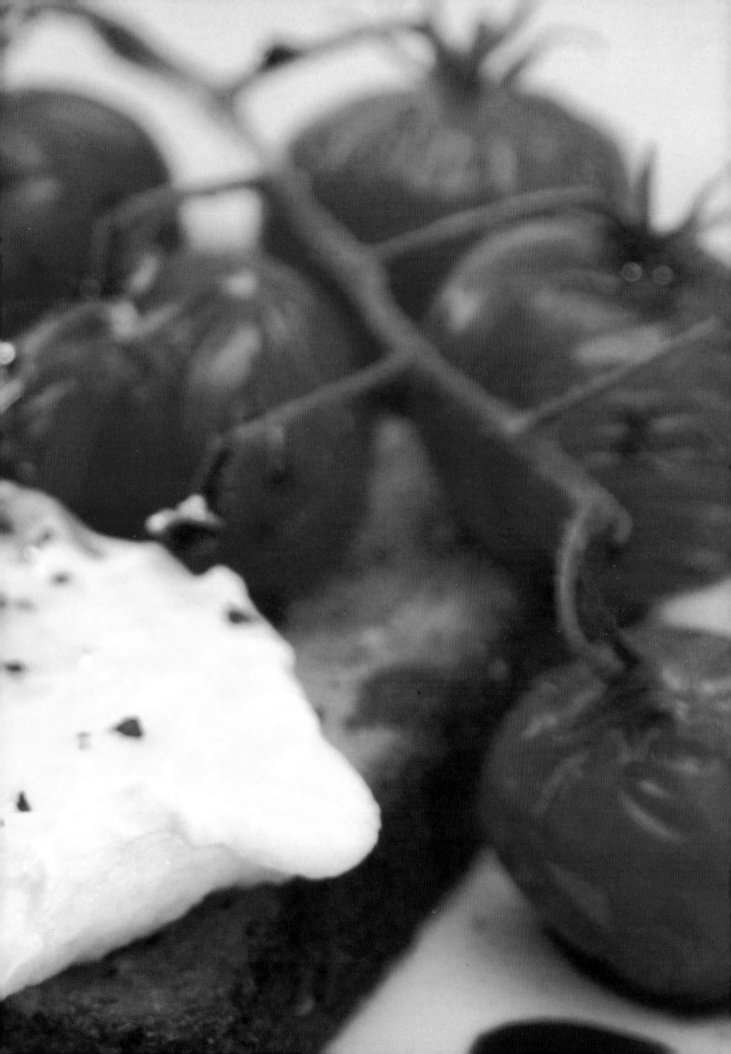

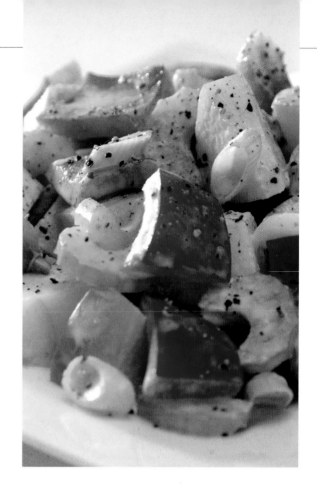

Healthy eating has become a hot topic in recent years, with a growing number of people showing real concerns about what they are eating. A considerable rise in food- and diet-related ailments and diseases is partly responsible for this. However, food scares and various unethical food-production practices have also played a part as 'extras' are added to our food – either at source or during production – which, given the chance, many of us would rather not be consuming. In addition to this, we have developed eating habits that, in the long run, could be doing us more harm than good.

# The trappings of convenience food

So often today we lead such busy lives that we find ourselves reaching for ready-prepared foods, convinced that we don't have time to cook anything else. We are drawn to these foods, which are highly processed and often so refined that much of the natural goodness is lost. Convenience foods tend to supply little by way of fibre or naturally occurring vitamins and minerals. Another disadvantage is that these foods are often loaded with fat, sugar and salt. If eaten regularly, it is possible almost to get hooked on the high sugar and fat content. The taste buds soon become used to this sort of taste and so will not appreciate natural, unprocessed foods.

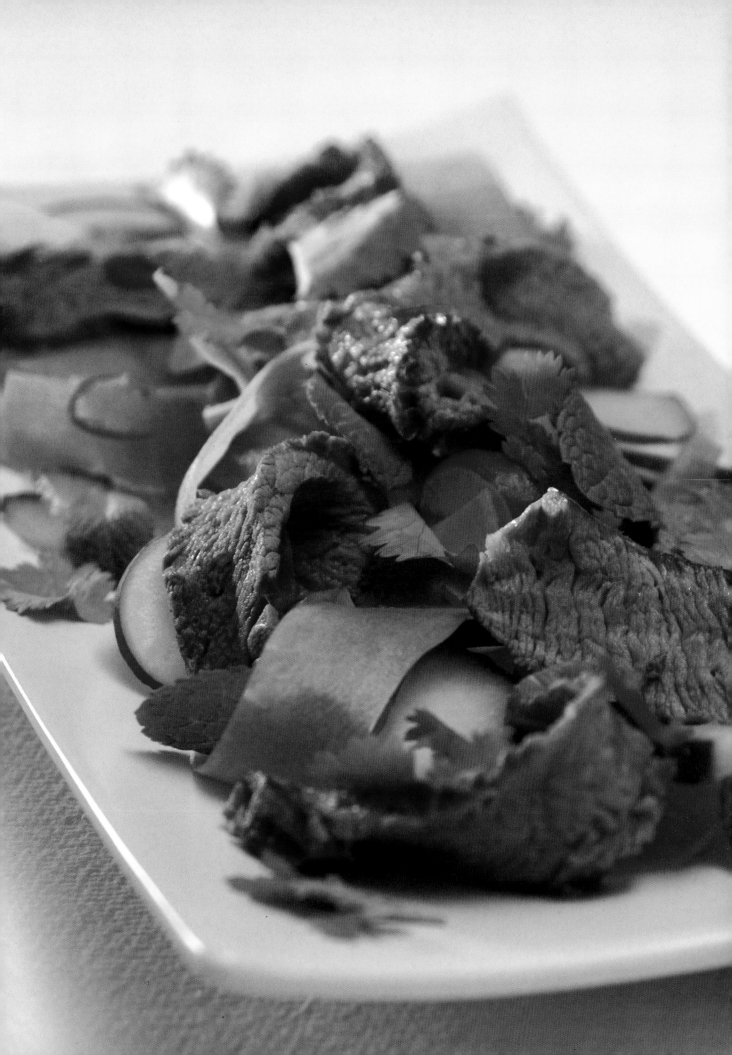

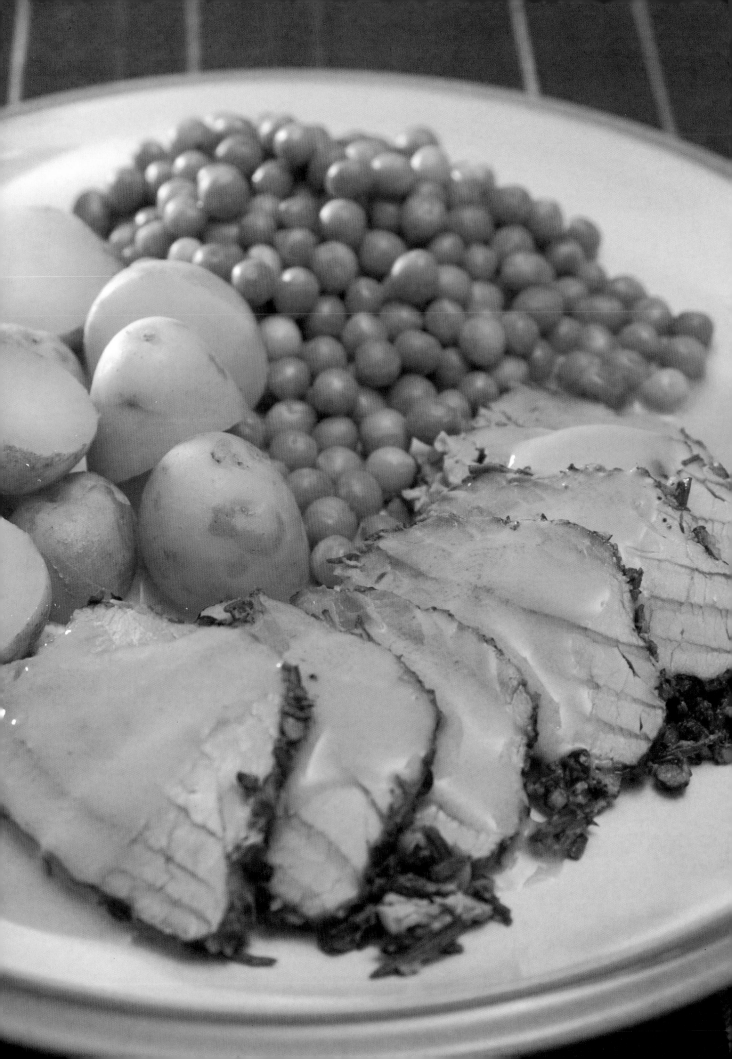

## All meat and no veg

The government has long been running a campaign to encourage us to eat more fruit and vegetables. Previous generations would have been surprised by this. Years ago meals consisted of meat, potatoes and at least two vegetables. And the vegetables and potatoes would have been in much larger portions than the meat because meat was very expensive. However, as we have become wealthier and farming methods have changed, we tend to eat in a very different way to our grandparents. Eating meat two or even three or four times a day – and in much larger portions – is now the norm for many people, and often not accompanied by any sort of vegetable. At first this would have been something that only the rich could afford, but which everyone aspired to. As meat became cheaper, it became accessible for the masses. No longer is meat eked out with vegetables and potatoes; instead meat is in abundance and vegetables are low on the list.

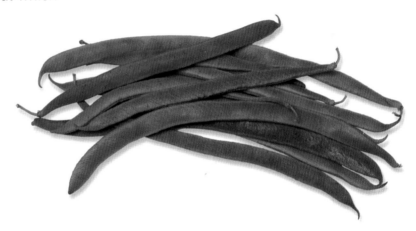

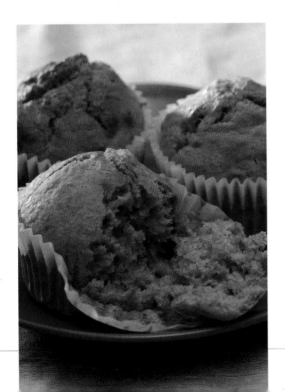

## Snacking

Our diets have changed dramatically in other ways too. In years gone by there would not have been the vast range of foods available today to snack on. People tended to eat three to four meals per day with little or nothing in between. This could be because the food was much more wholesome and so sustained appetites for longer, and perhaps it was also cultural, as people were not surrounded by advertisements of one sort or another trying to tempt them.

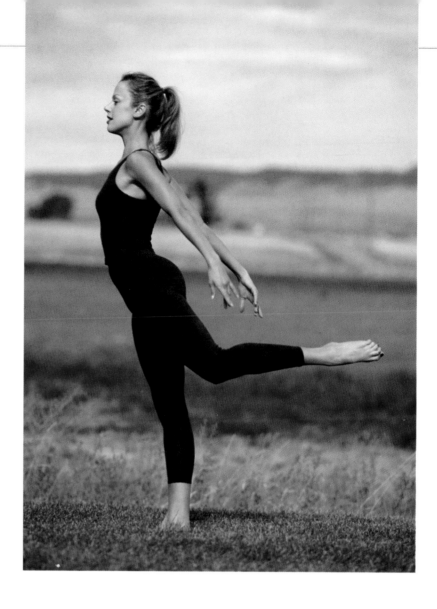

# Time for change

With a little effort, however, and a bit more thought, you can improve your diet, and subsequently your health, in a mere matter of weeks. One way to improve your diet is to opt for organic produce when it is available and affordable. This is an increasingly popular option for many people and is probably why the production of organic foods has been one of the fastest-growing industries to emerge in recent years. Supermarkets are stocking more and more organic produce, as well as quite an extensive range of whole foods that previously you would have had to obtain from a health food shop.

Another way to be more aware of what you are eating is, of course, by preparing it yourself. Making your own food not only guarantees freshness, but also allows you to control the quantities of fat, sugar and salt that you eat. Furthermore, home cooking eliminates preservatives and additives that are often contained in ready-prepared foods. Cooking is a life skill we should all possess – after all it produces the fuel that feeds our bodies. However, cooking does not have to be difficult in order for it to do us good. In fact, very long and complicated recipes can sometimes be the ones that are not so healthy! Perhaps advertising has persuaded you that anything quick and easy must come out of a packet, tin or jar. But this is not the case, and by experimenting in the kitchen, preferably when you are not under pressure from a starving family, a tight time schedule or a rumbling tummy, you will soon gain enough confidence and experience to be able to put a healthy meal together in the same time that it would take to cook that ready meal.

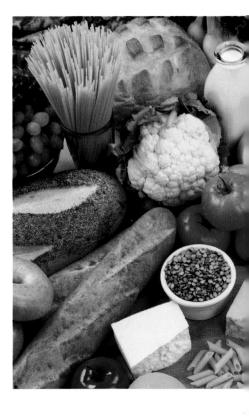

And when it comes to snacking, just remember that snacks do not have to be calorific, processed products. The range of snack foods available in supermarkets has been extended to include things like rice cakes, which you can eat as they are or with a topping of your choice, and one-portion cans of fruit in fruit juice. Another great snack is homemade popcorn – just remember to add only the tiniest sprinkle of sugar if you are having it sweetened. If you do not have time on your side, you can always grab a handful of dried apricots, banana chips, sunflower or pumpkin seeds, or, of course, a piece of fresh fruit.

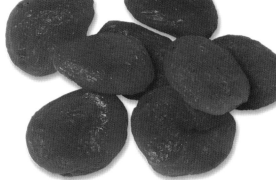

## All pain, no gain?

Unfortunately the phrase 'healthy eating' has connotations of pain rather than pleasure for some people. Even the word 'diet' is seen as something that is short term and restrictive – something that you can't wait to finish. 'Healthy' and 'diet' are two words that we should learn to look at in a more positive light. Thoughts of unappetising meals that are high in fibre and lacking in flavour generally lead people to give up before they have made a good start. Healthy eating really doesn't have to be like this, as this book should help you to see. Vegetables and fruits can be the basis of so many aspects of your everyday diet: salads, stews, casseroles, stir-fries and snacks, and by adding plenty of natural flavourings from herbs and spices you can significantly reduce the amount of salt in your diet.

The greatest challenge will be trying to break old habits. Don't give yourself unrealistic expectations – it is unfair and soul-destroying to try to make the transition from your previous daily regime to any sort of new one in just a matter of days – but if you can improve over a matter of weeks, and each week increase the positives and reduce the negatives, you are much more likely to succeed. And if you have a day when you achieve nothing positive in your new healthy eating regime, never mind – it is good that you are even aware of it, so just start again tomorrow, but do not give up.

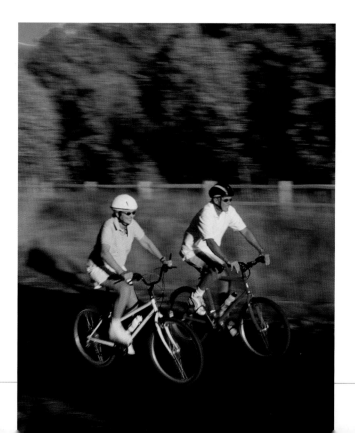

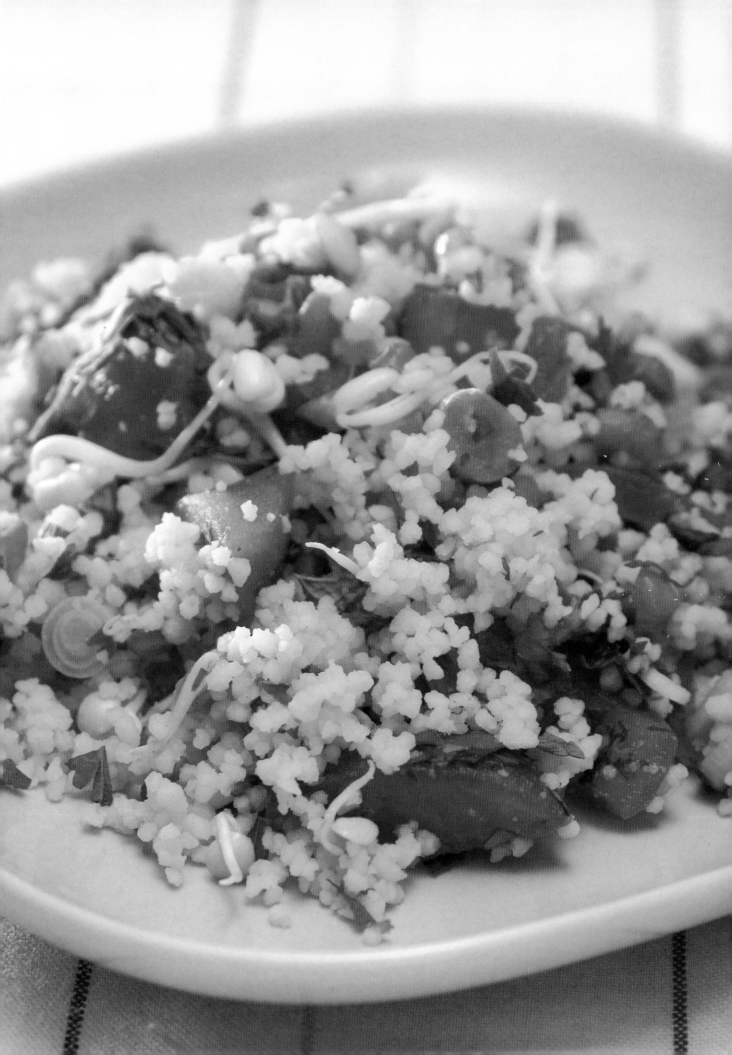

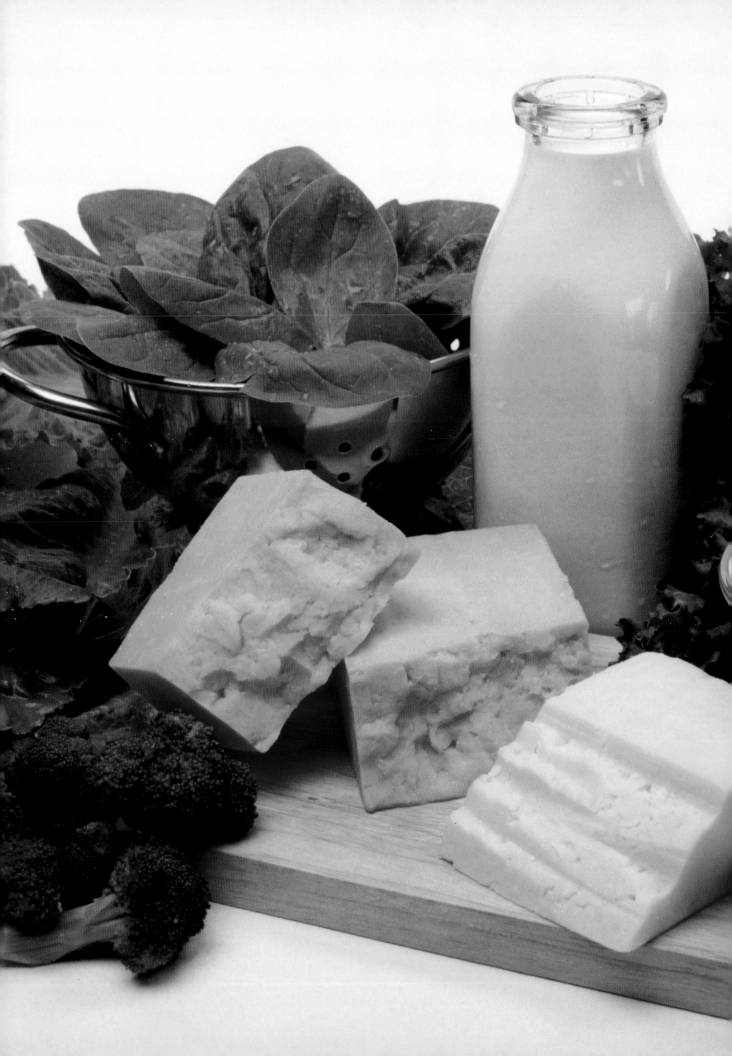

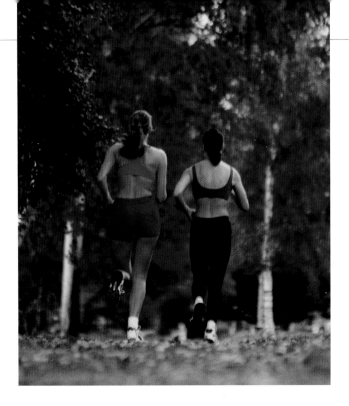

# A good model

Various studies have been carried out recently regarding the French and their diet. Considering their reputation for fine foods, which includes many full-fat cheeses, croissants, foie gras and creams, plus the fact that France is home to the gâteau, it is easy to imagine that they might all be suffering from obesity, amongst other things. This, however, is not the case, and after much analysis several factors seem to explain this. The first is that, although they continue to eat foods that are highly calorific or full fat (something that has been a part of their dietary tradition for many years), they eat them only in moderation. Furthermore, they have not replaced these foods with 'low-calorie' or 'low-fat' alternatives that have been manufactured and processed. Secondly, they are a nation that takes mealtimes seriously, treating them primarily as big family occasions. Lunch and supper are still meals that are eaten as a group, in a leisurely fashion, and at the table. They are not squeezed in between one activity and the next, or bolted down on the move. Each meal is given the importance it deserves – after all this is the fuel your body runs on. Both markets and shops stock fresh, seasonal, often local produce, and shopping for it is as much a social occasion as it is a necessity. Good food does not have to mean a lot of fuss or preparation. A piece of grilled steak with fresh herbs served with beans, baby carrots and new potatoes sounds fancy but depends on quality and freshness and needs minimal cooking or preparation. If a family wants a more instant meal the butcher supplies ready-prepared but home-cooked foods. As far as I am aware low-cost, large-sized foods are not such a phenomenon. People are much more interested in having fresh, good quality produce, even if it means smaller portions.

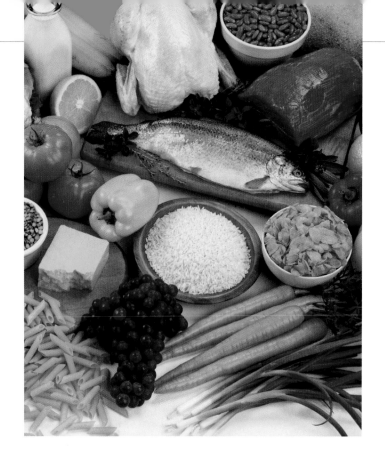

# Improving our eating habits

- Give a little more thought to what you eat, taking into account the fact that it is better to have seasonal, good-quality food in smaller portions. For example, several slices of highly processed white bread may not satisfy you, but one or two slices of a good wholewheat bread will keep your hunger at bay for much longer. It will also have added health benefits.

- Eat a little more slowly and think about what you are doing, rather than eating as you do something else. This ensures that you have time to chew your food properly, which will also help to prevent overeating, while lessening the risk of digestive problems. Take time to enjoy your food, chew it properly and relax.

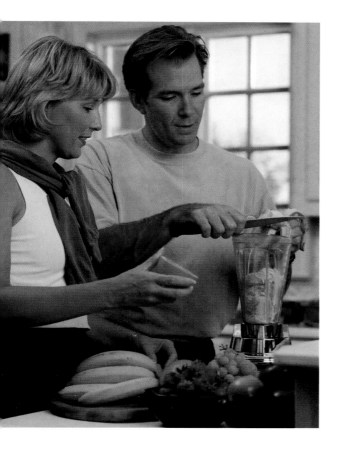

- Be imaginative and varied in your choice of foods. By being adventurous in what you eat you are probably less likely to overeat or become bored with your food. Some dieticians recommend we eat a 'rainbow diet' and I think this is a perfect way of summing it up in the simplest form. Different coloured fruits and vegetables provide us with different minerals and vitamins as do meats, fish, diary products, grains, pulses, and so on.

- Try always to buy the best that you can afford, aiming for quality rather than quantity. Check for freshness. Generally with fruit and vegetables, the skin should be firm and bright with no signs of damage or bruising. If they are looking limp, wrinkled or 'tired' don't buy them.

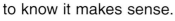

- Buy seasonal produce if you can. The difference in flavour is often well worth the wait. You only have to think of the first new season English strawberries and the ones you might buy in late November, to know it makes sense.

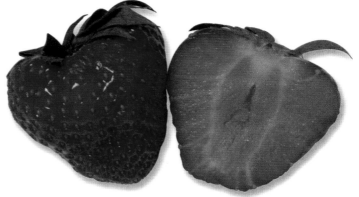

# A balanced diet

When it comes to building a balanced diet, there are five main food groups.

## Fruit and vegetables

Fruit and vegetables are rich in so much that is essential for our wellbeing that it is hardly surprising we need to be eating more of them. And with the huge variety now available to us, we really should have little or no excuse. Although fresh is always best, we can also choose from frozen and canned as well as dried. If you are opting for the canned variety, check the ingredients list to make sure nothing else has been added. Years ago, canned foods were packed in water with sugar or salt added. Although this is often still the case, many brands also offer a no-added-sugar or -salt version, so check the label. Fruit and vegetables are good sources of vitamins and minerals, some of which cannot be stored in the body and need to be eaten on a daily basis. They are an excellent source of fibre, which is vital for a healthy diet. Versatility and variety should be your aim, so eat as many different sorts as you can in order to benefit from them as much as possible. We should eat at least five portions of fruit and vegetables every day (some countries are now recommending 9–10).

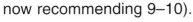

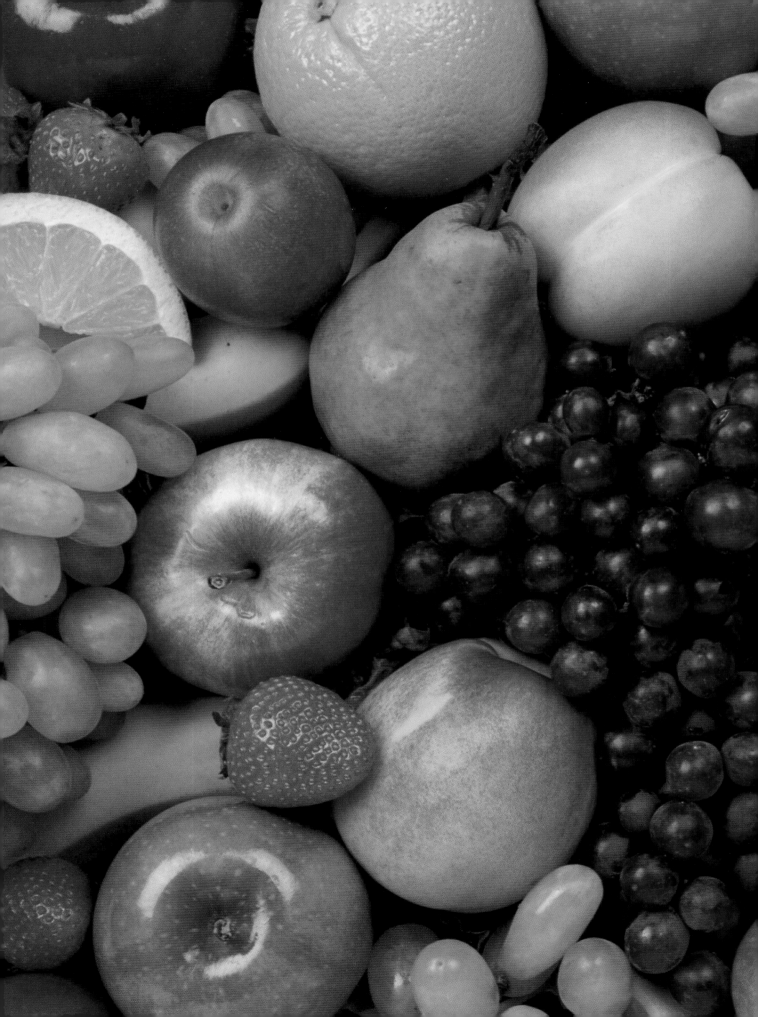

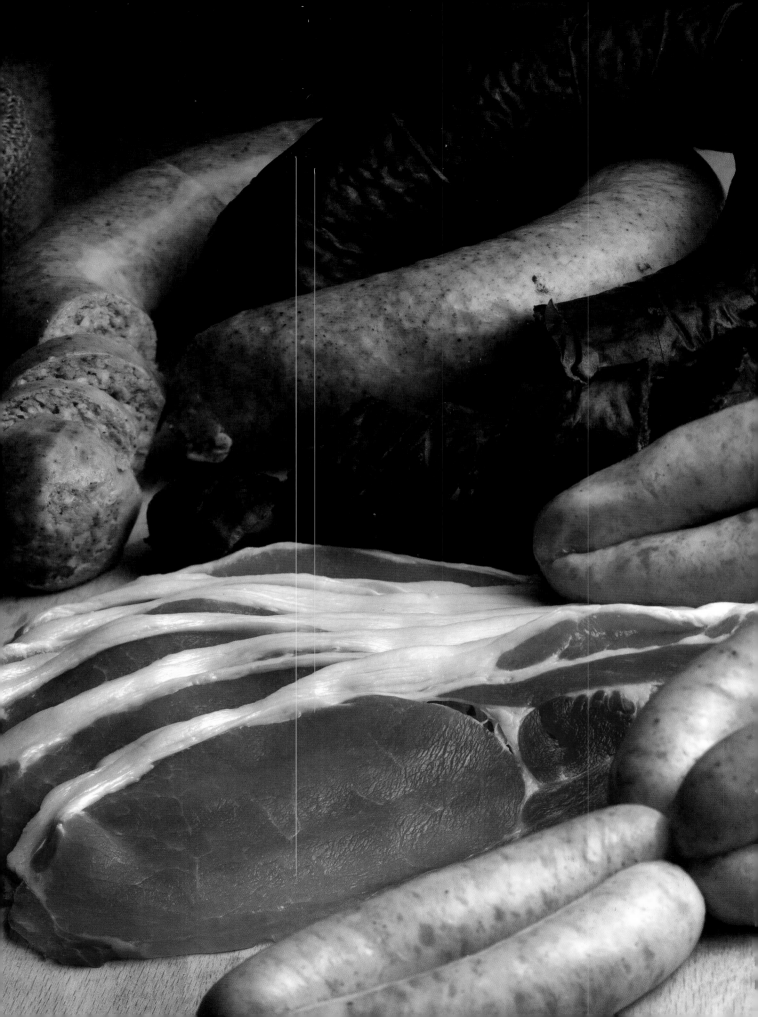

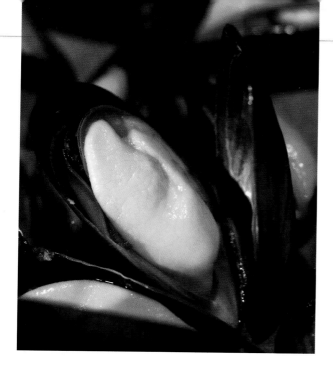

## Meat and Fish

These are good sources of protein, fat, some B vitamins and minerals (mostly iron and zinc). Look out for lean cuts of meat – chicken and pork tend to be leaner than lamb and beef, depending on the cut. Fish supplies protein and B vitamins as well as vitamins A, D and F (depending on which variety you are eating). It also contains unsaturated fats, which are good for us. Oily fish provides omega-3 fatty acids, which are important for the health of your heart, amongst other things. Quick to cook, especially when prepared by a fishmonger, fish is probably the original fast food.

Women need approximately 45g of protein a day. This requirement should be increased if you lead a very active life or are pregnant or breastfeeding. Men need approximately 55g, which should also be increased if you are active. Generally we tend to eat more protein than we need each day, which can cause weight gain.

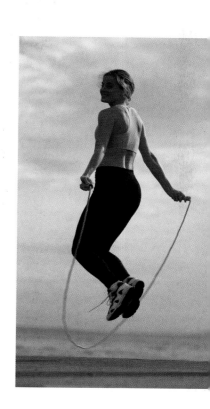

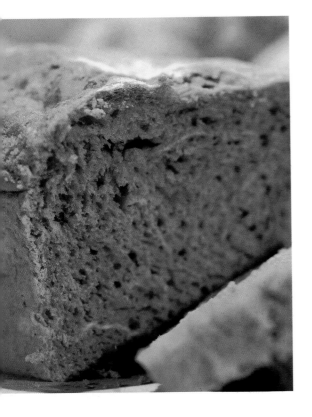

## carbohydrates

Our main and most important source of energy is carbohydrate, which is mainly provided by plant foods. There are three main types of carbohydrate: simple sugars, complex carbohydrates or starches, and dietary fibre. Of the three, complex carbohydrates are now known to be positively beneficial to our health and should be included on a daily basis. They are found in bread, pasta, rice, barley, millet, buckwheat and rye. The World Health Organization (WHO) recommends a diet that consists of 50–70 per cent complex carbohydrates. Wholegrain foods or unrefined foods are high in dietary fibre as are fruit, both fresh and dried, and vegetables. Ensuring you eat plenty of dietary fibre is now known to be a good safeguard against many digestive ailments and can even help protect you against cancer of the colon.

Simple sugars are found in fruit, milk and ordinary sugar. Refined sources of sugar are not good to include in your diet as they provide none of the fibre, vitamins or minerals and are the main cause of dental decay.

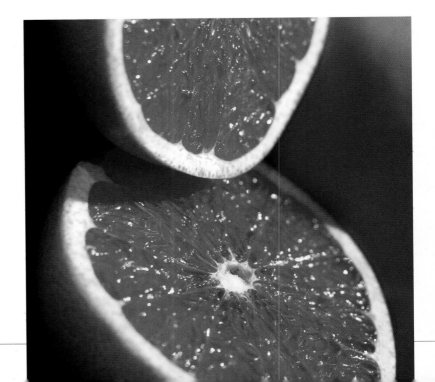

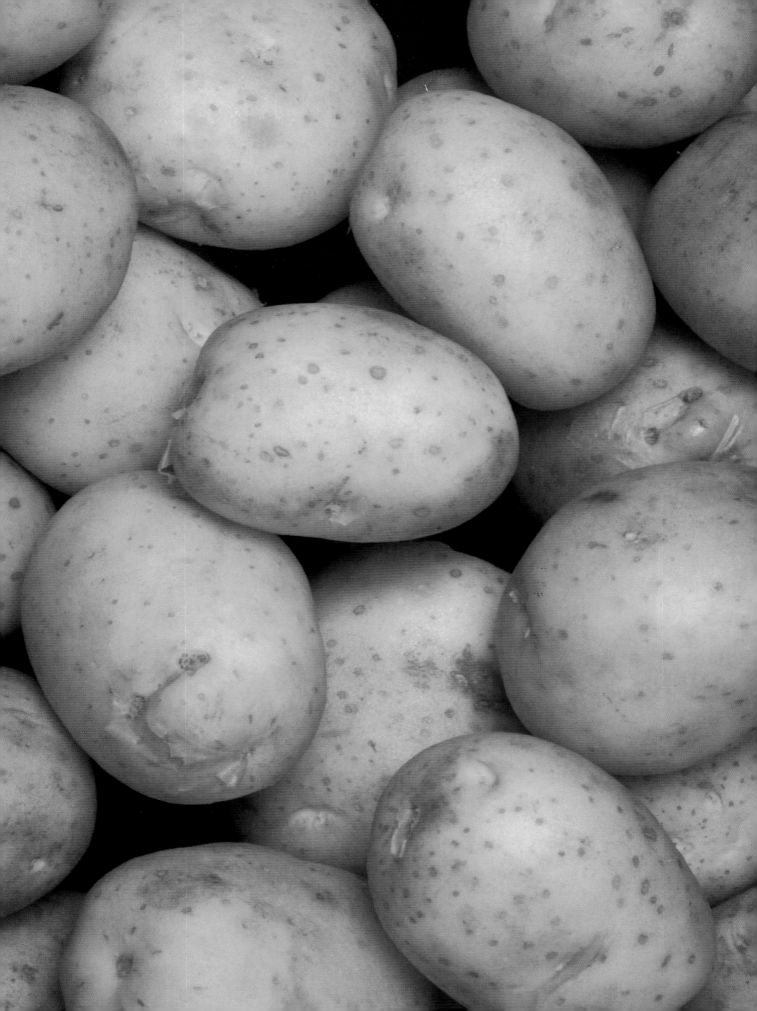

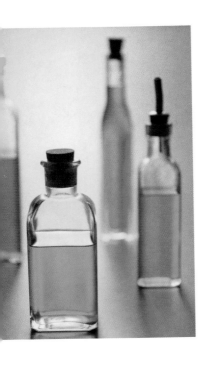

## Fats and Oils

Fats and oils get bad press but they are also essential in a balanced diet. The important thing is to eat the right sort and not to excess. They are necessary for the manufacture of hormones and also as a carrier for some vitamins and to help keep our tissues in good repair. Fats are either saturated or non saturated, with non-saturated fats catagorised as being either mono-unsaturated or polyunsaturated. Animal fats tend to be saturated and a high intake of these can lead to raised blood cholesterol and a higher risk of heart disease. Our bodies need a little fat (preferably mono-unsaturated or polyunsaturated) each day to ensure that certain dietary vitamins are properly absorbed into our systems. Mono-unsaturated oils include olive oil and peanut oil and polyunsaturated oils include sesame seed oil and sunflower oil.

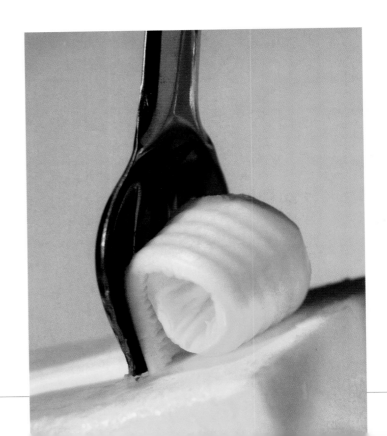

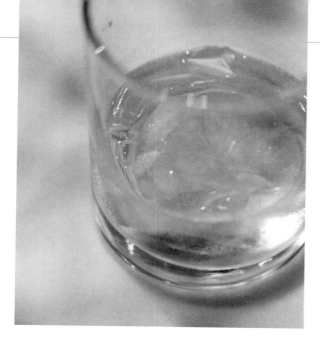

## Water

We all know that we should drink more water, but it is not until you start keeping a record of how many glasses you drink a day that you will see how near or far you are from your goal. You really need to aim for about 2 to 3 litres (4 to 5 pints) per day. This can seem daunting, but if you carry a bottle of water with you as you go about your day, you can keep sipping at it, which will help. If you only drink when you are thirsty you may already be dehydrated. It is better to drink a little and often, rather than leaving it until you are thirsty and then drinking lots. Drinking the right amount of water each day will go some way towards helping you increase your energy levels. (The body is made up of over 60 per cent water, which is constantly being used to keep us fit and healthy, and needs constant replenishing.) Tea and coffee are mild diuretics so should not be included in your daily water intake. Try to limit yourself to two or three cups per day. Herbal teas are fine, however, as is adding a slice of lemon or ginger to a mug of hot water. There runs a constant debate as to whether the water you drink should be still or sparkling. It is probably more important to drink the right amount and you can possibly try a mix of the two. Buying a water filter that fits in the fridge door is a good idea, as it will not only save you money in the long run but will also mean that you are doing something towards helping the environment by keeping plastic and glass production down.

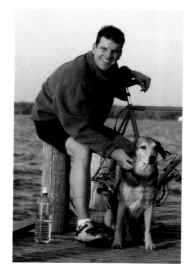

# using this book

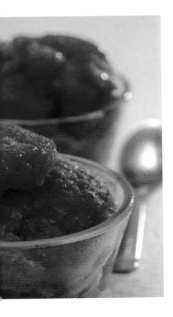

*Healthy Meals* offers 100 recipes for an improved diet. I have tried to use natural foods and to steer away from foods that have been 'reduced' i.e. low fat or low calorie. With naturally produced foods, we know much more about both their advantages and disadvantages than we do about the processed alternatives. The recipes do not focus purely on ingredients, but also on the way foods are cooked. Steaming, stir-frying, and cooking as part of a stew or casserole are healthy and tasty alternatives to shallow or deep-frying. This book does not promise to make you lose weight or to transform your life, but it should show you just how easy it is to eat a healthy diet that is tasty and full of flavour without expending too much effort.

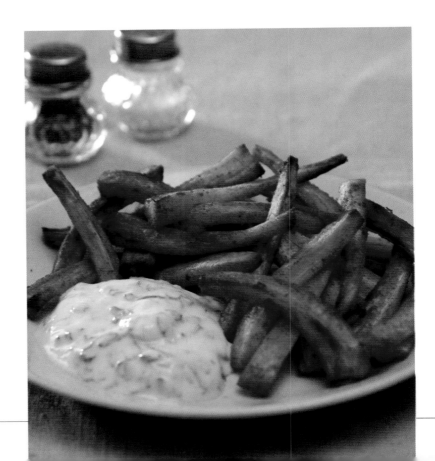

# Tips for Successful Cooking

- Use metric or imperial measurements only; do not mix the two.

- Use measuring spoons: 1 tsp = 5ml; 1 tbsp = 15ml

- All spoon measurements are level unless otherwise stated.

- All eggs are medium unless otherwise stated.

- Recipes using raw or lightly cooked eggs should not be given to babies, pregnant women, the very old or anyone suffering from or recovering from an illness.

- The cooking times are an approximate guide only. If you are using a fan oven reduce the cooking time according to the manufacturer's instructions.

- Ovens should be preheated to the required temperature.

- Fruit and vegetables should be washed before use.

Please note – most of the recipes have ingredients listed for a number of servings. If the recipe includes servings for two and four people, for example, it will show how much to add for two people, with the amount for four people in brackets, e.g. 2 tbsp (4 tbsp).

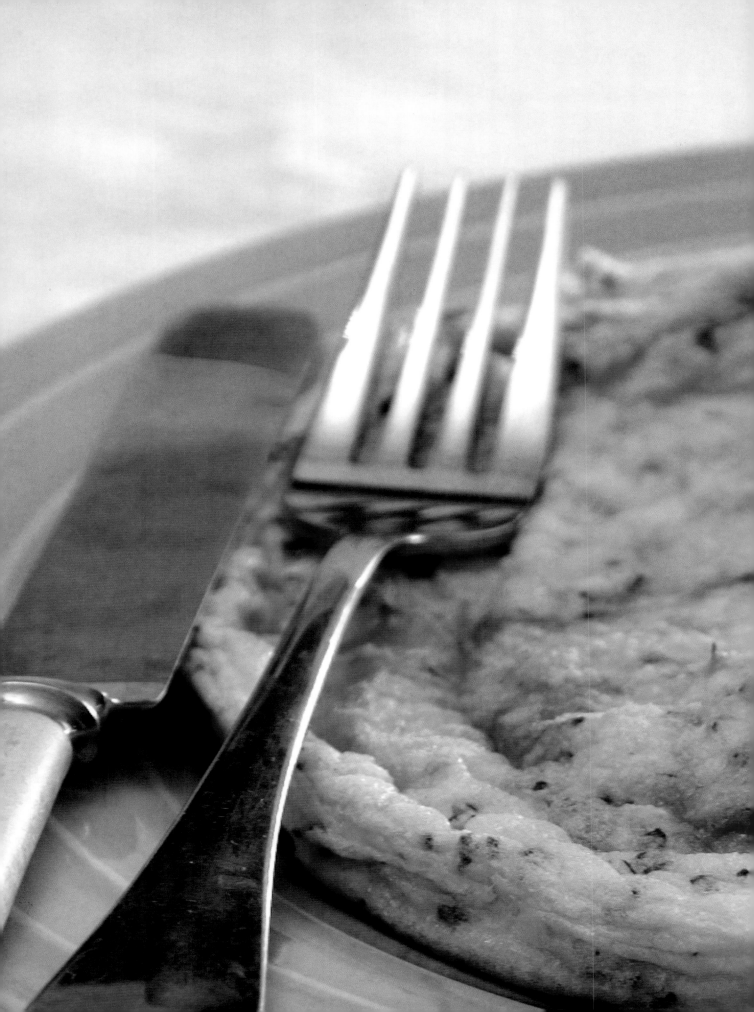

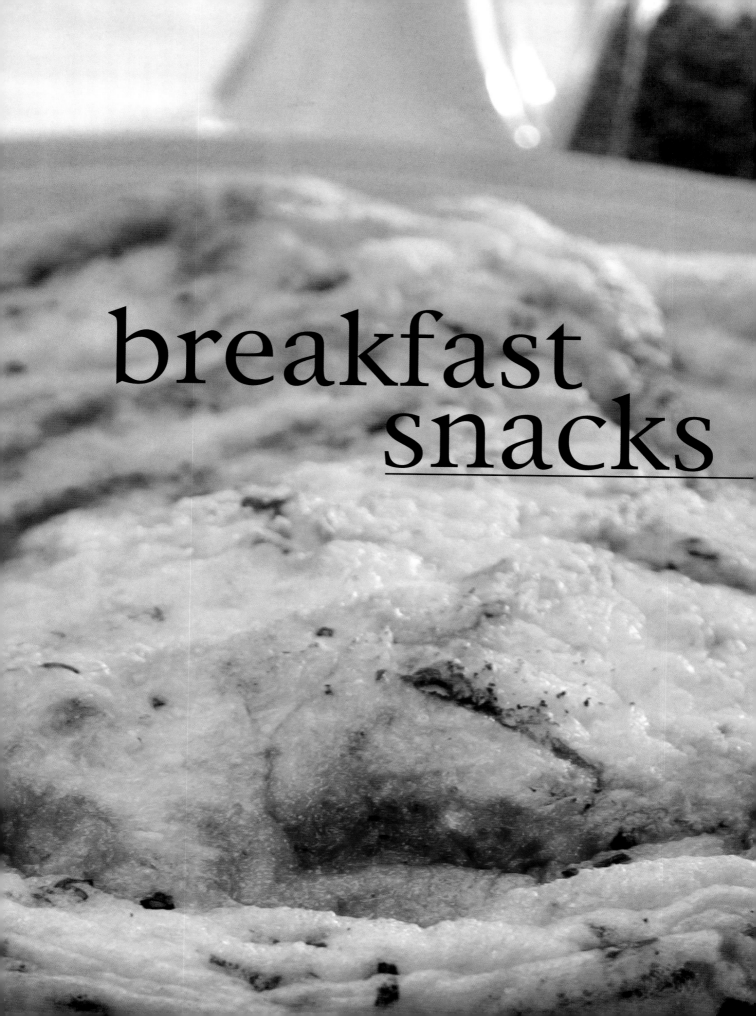

breakfast
snacks

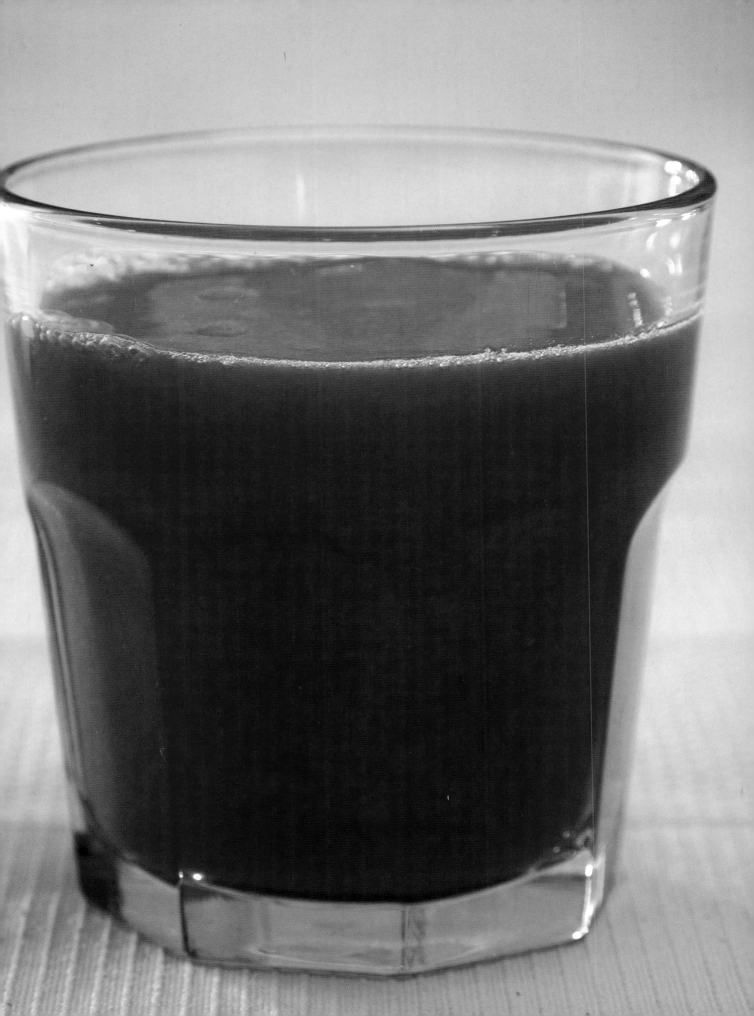

# Super Boost Juice

*Family Favourite*

Beetroot is high in vitamins and minerals, while ginger has a wide range of benefits, including aiding digestion and circulation and stimulating the liver. Apples and carrots are both excellent sources of vitamins C and A respectively.

### Serves 2

**1 small beetroot**
**4 eating apples**
**4 large carrots**
**1cm/½in fresh ginger**

### Serves 4

**2 small beetroot**
**8 eating apples**
**8 large carrots**
**2.5cm/1in fresh ginger**

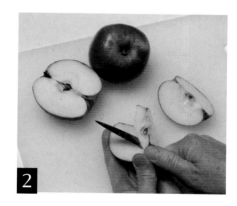

1 Peel the beetroot and cut into chunks. It might be best to wear rubber gloves as the beetroot can stain your hands.

2 Quarter and core the apples.

3 Trim and peel the carrots.

4 Peel the ginger. It is easiest to do this by scraping a teaspoon over the skin of the ginger. The skin will come away easily with little waste.

5 Now process all the prepared fruit and vegetables through a juicer.

6 Stir and serve immediately, adding ice if desired.

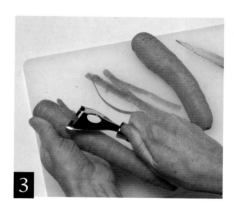

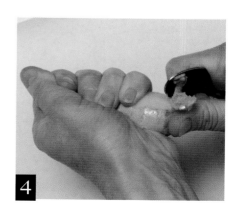

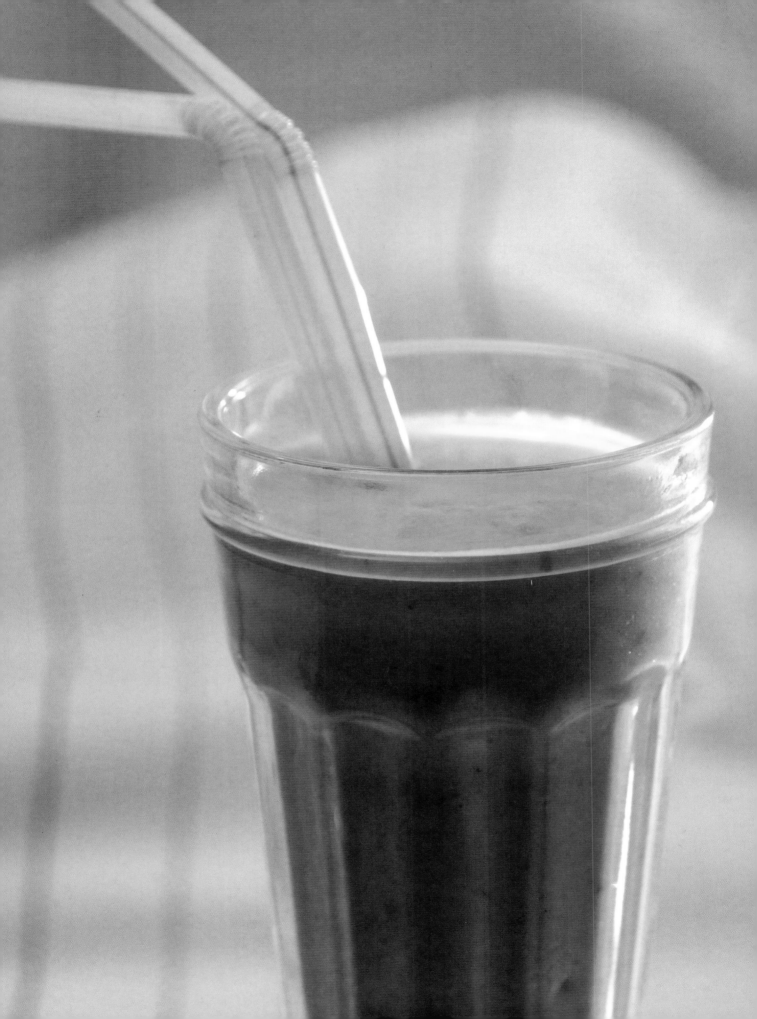

# Mango & Raspberry Smoothie

*Children's Choice*

Made in minutes and so good, you might drink it all!

## Serves 2

**1 small mango**
**100g/4oz raspberries, fresh**
**or frozen and defrosted**
**600ml/1pt semi-skimmed**
**milk**
**2 tsp honey, optional**
**ice cubes**

## Serves 4

**1 large mango**
**200g/7oz raspberries, fresh**
**or frozen and defrosted**
**1.2l/2pt semi-skimmed milk**
**4 tsp honey, optional**
**ice cubes**

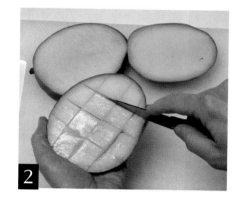

1 The stone of a mango is quite large and fat. The best way to get as much of the flesh as possible is to cut the mango in two thick slices either side of the stone.

2 Cut the flesh on these slices almost through to the skin in a criss-cross pattern.

3 Press the skin upwards. The pieces of flesh should pop up, making it easy to get a small, sharp knife between flesh and skin, producing small cubes of mango flesh.

4 Trim the skin from the mango and then trim away as much of the flesh as you can from around the stone.

5 In a food processor or liquidiser, combine the mango flesh and raspberries and blend until smooth. Add the milk, honey if using and a large handful of ice cubes and blend again. Serve immediately.

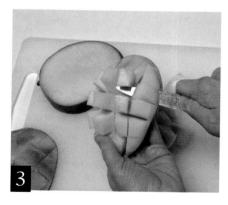

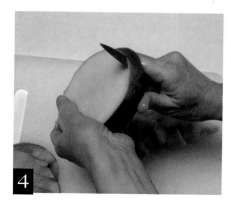

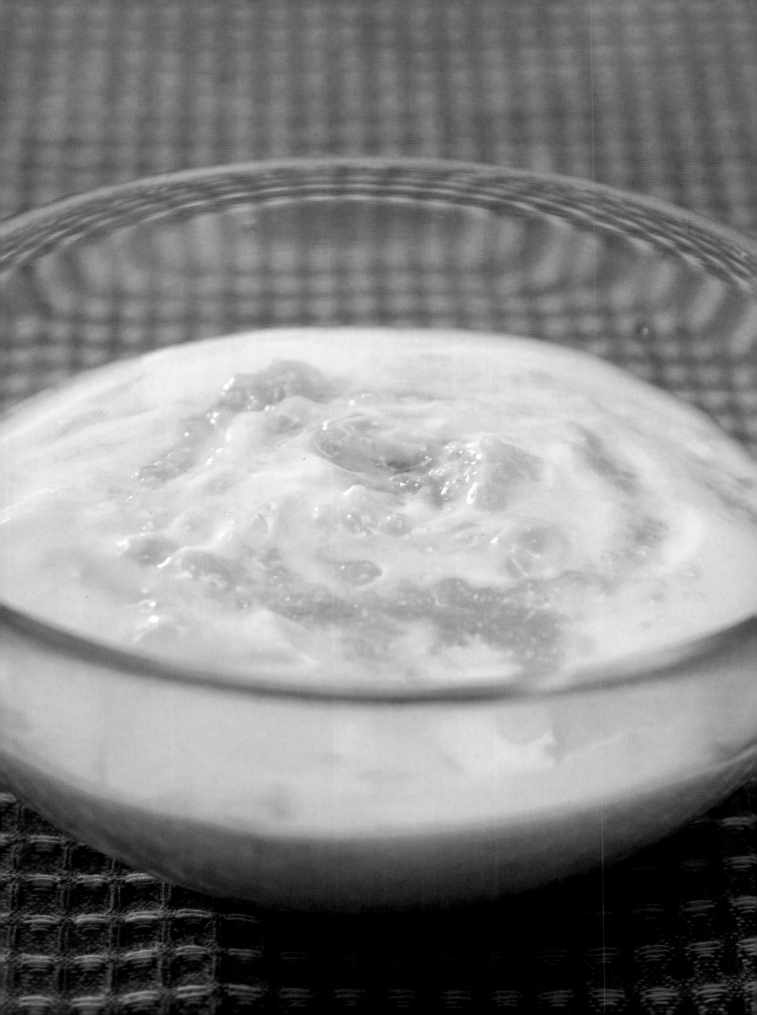

# Apricot & Yoghurt

## Children's Choice

Apricots are an excellent source of iron and potassium and yoghurt is rich in calcium.

### Serves 2

**50g/2oz dried ready-to-eat apricots**
**1 orange**
**1 tsp honey**
**250ml/9fl oz plain yoghurt**

### Serves 4

**100g/4oz dried ready-to-eat apricots**
**1 large orange**
**2 tsp honey**
**500ml/18fl oz plain yoghurt**

1 Roughly chop the apricots and place them in a saucepan.

2 Wash the orange and dry thoroughly. Now finely grate the zest and add to the apricots. Halve the orange and squeeze the juice.

3 Add the juice, honey and 2 (4) tbsp water to the pan. Place over a gentle heat and cook, stirring from time to time. Bring gently to the boil. Remove from the heat and set to one side to cool. It is best to prepare to this point a day in advance.

4 When the apricot mixture is cold, place it in a food processor or blender and process briefly. If you prefer you can process the mixture until it is completely smooth but I think it is better with a bit of texture.

5 Place the yoghurt in a bowl and then add the apricot mixture. Now, using a large spoon, give the mixture one or two quick stirs to swirl the apricot through the yoghurt. Serve.

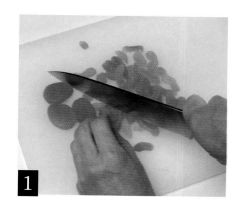

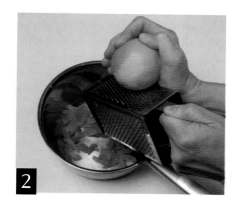

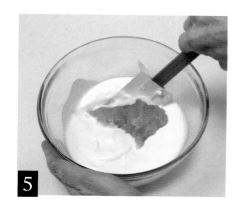

# Porridge

*Family Favourite*

Porridge is a great way to start the day, as it provides a slow-release carbohydrate that will keep you going until lunchtime. Oats are also good for helping to reduce bad cholesterol in the body.

*Serves 2*

**75g/3oz medium oatmeal**
**600ml/1pt semi-skimmed milk**
**3 tbsp Greek yoghurt**
**2 tbsp runny honey**

*Serves 4*

**175g/6oz medium oatmeal**
**1.2l/2pt semi-skimmed milk**
**6 tbsp Greek yoghurt**
**4 tbsp runny honey**

1 Place the oatmeal in a large saucepan and add the milk, whisking as you do so.

2 Cook over a gentle heat, stirring regularly to prevent lumps forming. Bring gently to the boil. The porridge will be starting to thicken at this point. Now reduce the heat and cook for a further 5 minutes.

3 Remove from the heat and divide between 2 (4) bowls. Divide the yoghurt evenly between the bowls and finish by topping with the honey. Serve.

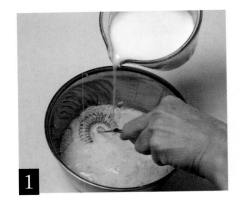

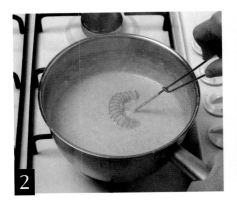

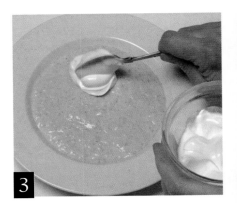

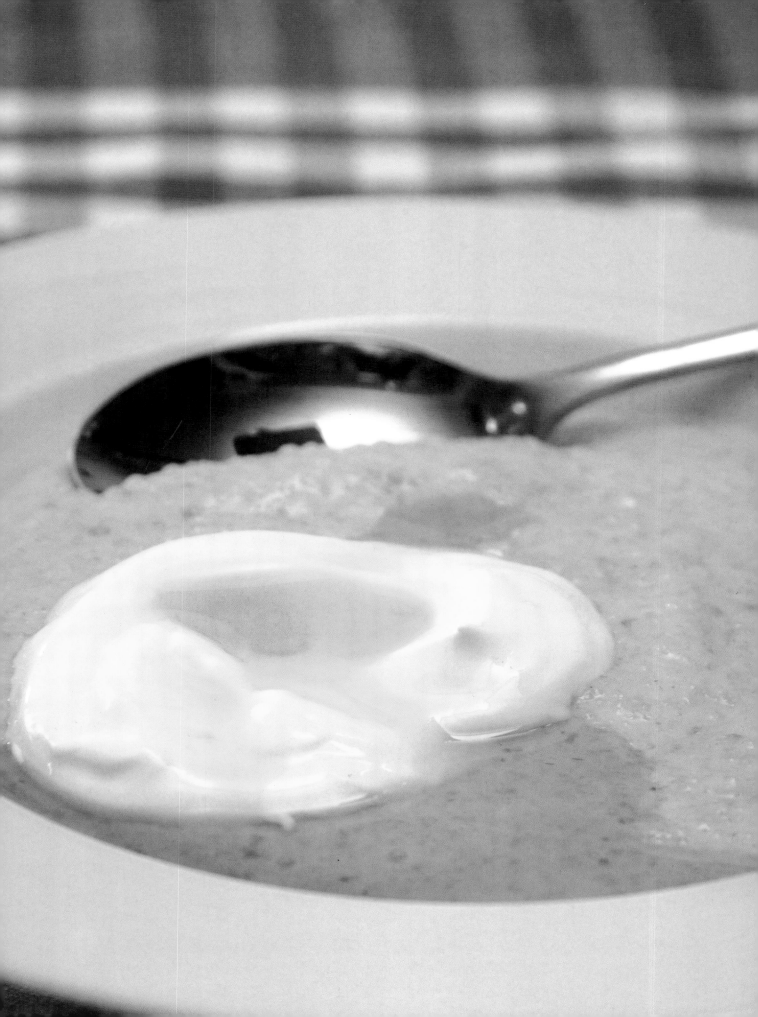

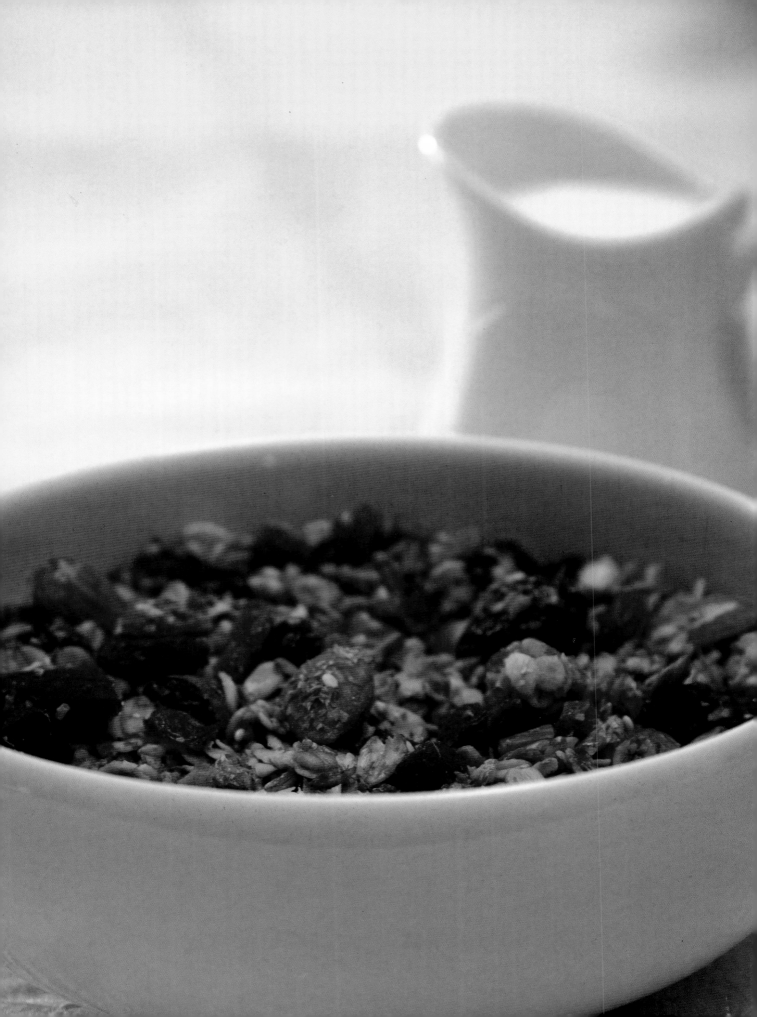

# Granola

## Children's Choice

By making your own cereal you can ensure that salt hasn't been added and that the sweetness level is not excessive. The combination of oats with seeds, nuts and dried fruits makes this a highly nutritious breakfast.

### Makes approximately 10 servings

**450g/1lb rolled oats**
**75g/3oz bran**
**100g/4oz sunflower seeds**
**25g/1oz sesame seeds**
**100g/4oz whole almonds**
**100ml/3½fl oz runny honey**
**100ml/3½fl oz sunflower oil**
**150g/5oz sultanas, raisins and dates, mixed**

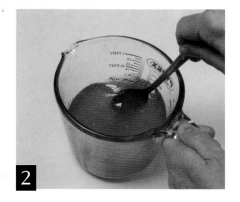

1 Preheat the oven to 180°C/350°F/Gas Mark 4. In a large mixing bowl, combine the oats, bran, sunflower and sesame seeds and mix well. Add the almonds.

2 Measure the honey into a measuring jug and then add 100ml/3½fl oz boiling water and stir well to mix. Now add the oil and stir again.

3 Pour this mixture over the oat and seed mixture, stirring well to mix. Spread the mixture over a large baking tray.

4 Bake in the oven for about 25 minutes, stirring the outside edges into the middle about 2–3 times, to ensure even cooking. Remove from the oven and stir in the dried fruits. Set to one side to cool fully. When cold, store in an airtight container and use as required.

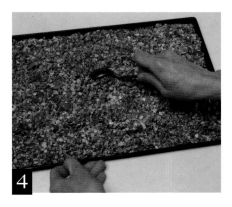

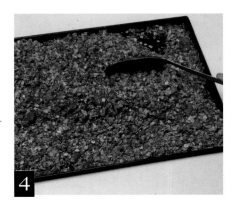

# Dried Fruit Salad

*Quick and Easy*

Dried fruits are high in fibre and rich in minerals, including iron. One serving counts as one to two portions of your daily five portions of fruit and vegetables.

### Serves 2

**200g/7oz mixed dried fruits (apple, pear, prune, fig, etc)**
**300ml/½pt apple juice**
**½ cinnamon stick**
**1½ star anise**
**½ tbsp runny honey**
**Greek yoghurt to serve**

### Serves 4

**400g/14oz mixed large dried fruits (apple, pear, prune, fig, etc)**
**600ml/1pt apple juice**
**1 cinnamon stick**
**3 star anise**
**1 tbsp runny honey**
**Greek yoghurt to serve**

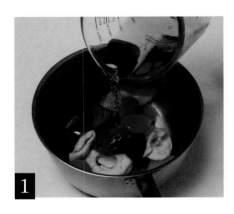

1 Place the dried fruits in a large saucepan and pour over the apple juice.

2 Add the cinnamon stick and star anise and bring gently to the boil, stirring from time to time.

3 Remove from the heat and stir in the honey. Cover and set to one side to cool. Before serving, remove the cinnamon and star anise and discard. Serve with Greek yoghurt if desired. Alternatively this can be served warm or even to accompany cereal or porridge.

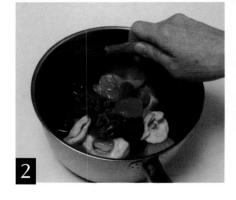

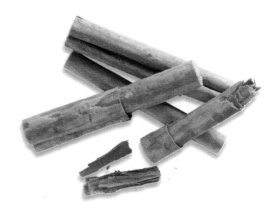

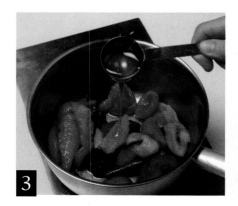

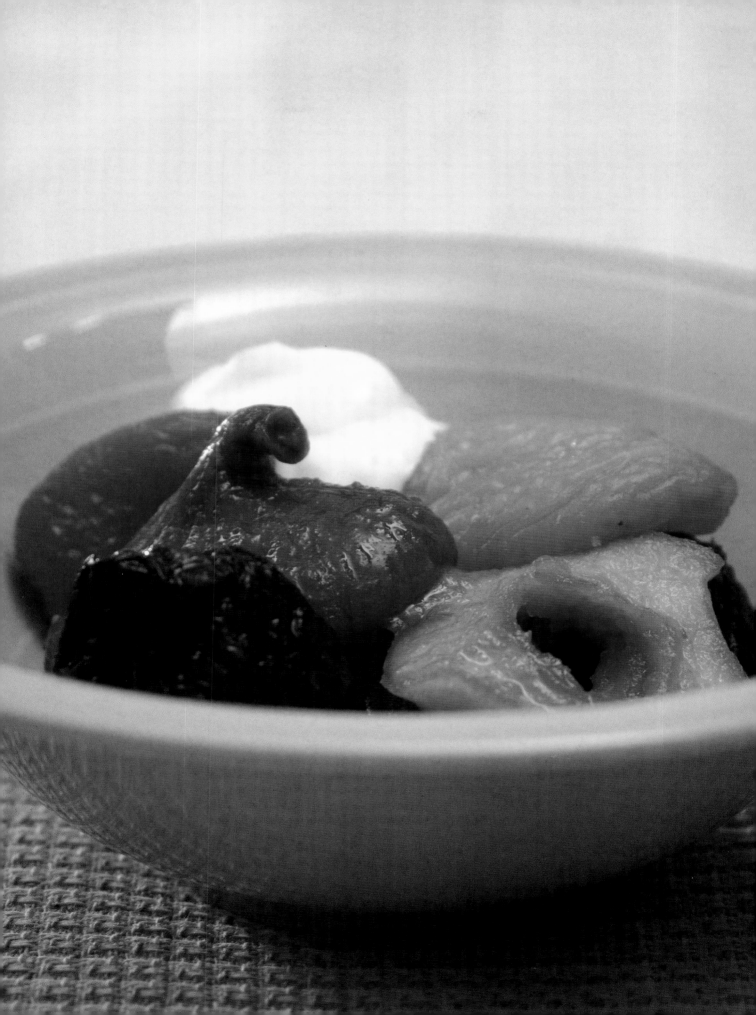

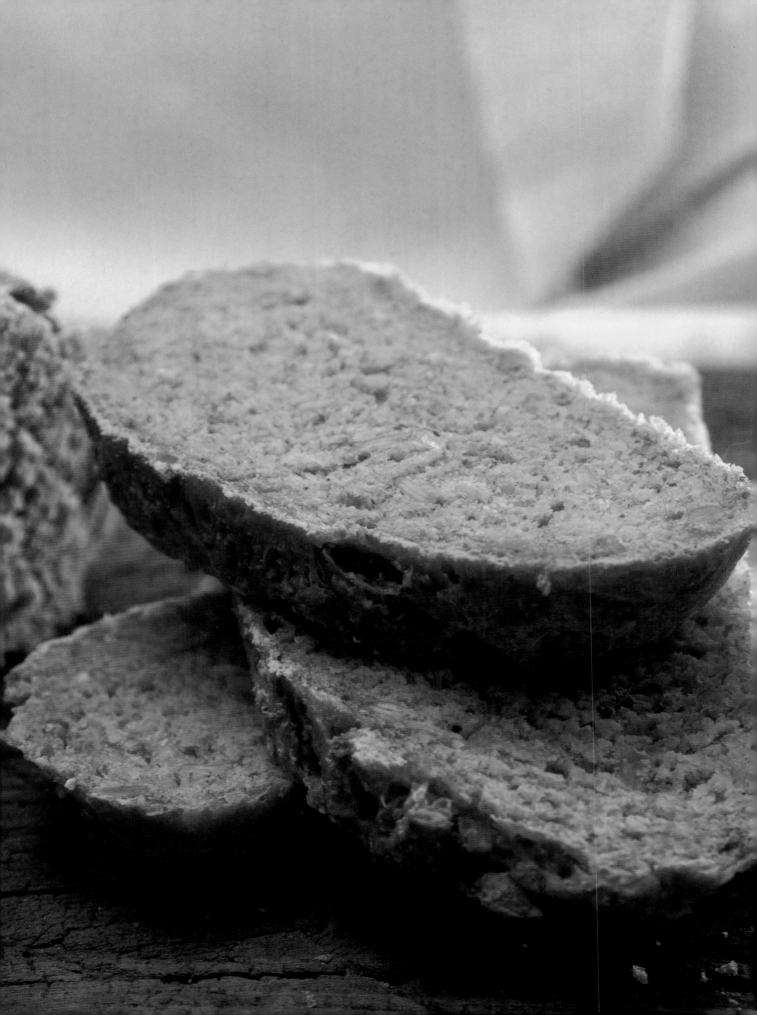

# Oat & Sunflower Bread

*Family Favourite*

Oats are good for helping to lower bad cholesterol as well as being good for your heart.

## Makes 1 loaf

**100g/4oz medium oatmeal**
**200g/7oz strong white flour**
**200g/7oz strong wholemeal flour**
**50g/2oz rolled oats**
**50g/2oz sunflower seeds**
**1 tsp salt**
**7g/¼oz easy-blend yeast**
**2 tbsp honey**
**1 tbsp sunflower oil**

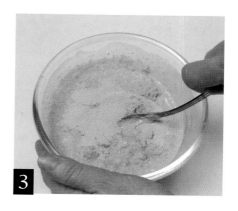

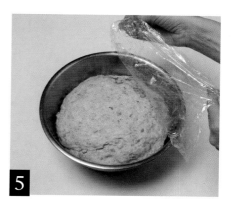

1 Place the oatmeal in a mixing bowl and cover with 300ml/½pt boiling water. Set to one side to soak, overnight.

2 Stir the white and wholemeal flours together. Add the rolled oats, sunflower seeds and salt and stir again.

3 Sprinkle the yeast over the soaked oatmeal and stir. Mix the honey into 150ml/¼pt tepid water along with the oil. Now add both the soaked oatmeal and the liquid to the flour mixture and mix well to form a dough, adding a little more tepid water if necessary.

4 Turn out onto a lightly floured surface and knead for approximately 10 minutes, until the dough becomes springy to the touch and is no longer sticky.

5 Return the dough to the mixing bowl and cover with a piece of lightly oiled cling film. Leave in a warm place until the dough has doubled in size.

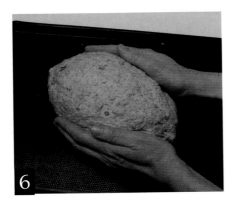

6 Remove the dough from the bowl and knead for 2–3 minutes. Now shape the dough into a long oval (or shape of your choice) and place on a lightly oiled baking sheet. Cover with lightly oiled cling film and leave in a warm place to rise once again.

7 Preheat the oven to 220°C/425°F/Gas Mark 7. When the dough has almost doubled in size, remove the cling film. Bake in the oven for 20 minutes then reduce the temperature to 190°C/375°F/Gas Mark 5 and bake for a further 15 minutes. Remove from the tin and cool on a wire rack. Serve.

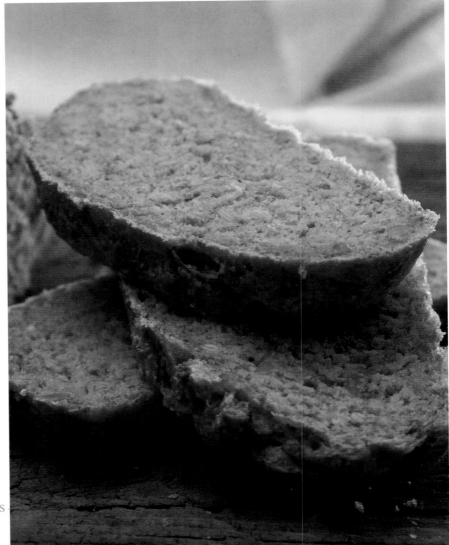

# Breakfast Bread

## Family Favourite

By making your own bread you can keep a better control over your sugar and salt intake, which is often high in ready-prepared foods. This bread is delicious warm or cold, and if it is a day or two old, just pop it in the toaster.

### Makes 1 loaf

**450g/1lb strong wholemeal flour**
**1 heaped tsp caraway seeds**
**7g/¼oz easy-blend yeast**
**1 tsp salt**
**100g/4oz walnuts, roughly chopped**
**100g/4oz dried sour cherries**
**1 tbsp sunflower oil**
**3 tbsp molasses**

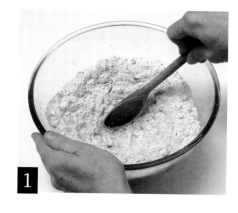

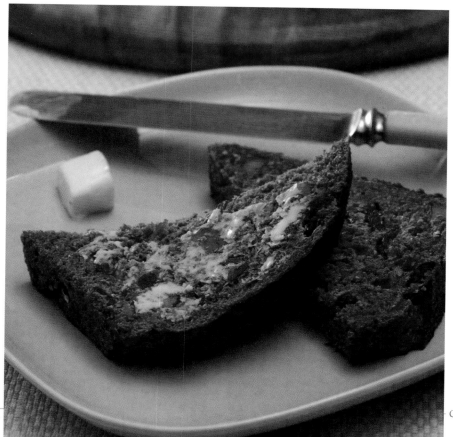

1  Place the flour in a large mixing bowl, add the caraway seeds and yeast and stir well to mix. Add the salt, walnuts and cherries and stir again. Make a well in the centre.

2  Measure 300ml/½pt tepid water. Add the sunflower oil and molasses and mix well. Pour this liquid into the flour mixture and stir quickly until the mixture starts to form a dough, adding a little more tepid water if necessary.

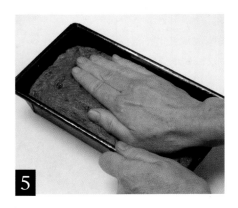

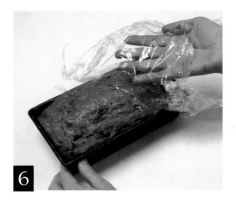

3 Turn out on to a lightly floured surface and knead for approximately 10 minutes, until the dough becomes springy to the touch and is no longer sticky.

4 Return the dough to the mixing bowl and cover with a piece of lightly oiled cling film. Leave in a warm place until the dough has doubled in size.

5 Remove the dough from the bowl and knead for 2–3 minutes. Lightly oil a 900g/2lb loaf tin and press the dough into the tin. Cover with lightly oiled cling film and leave in a warm place to rise once again.

6 Preheat the oven to 220°C/425°F/Gas Mark 7. When the dough has risen, remove the cling film. Bake in the oven for 20 minutes, then reduce the temperature to 190°C/375°F/Gas Mark 5 and bake for a further 15 minutes. Remove from the tin and cool on a wire rack. Serve.

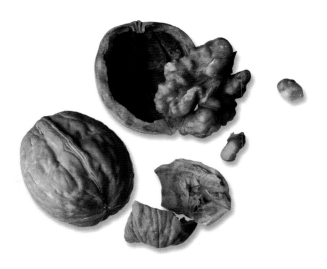

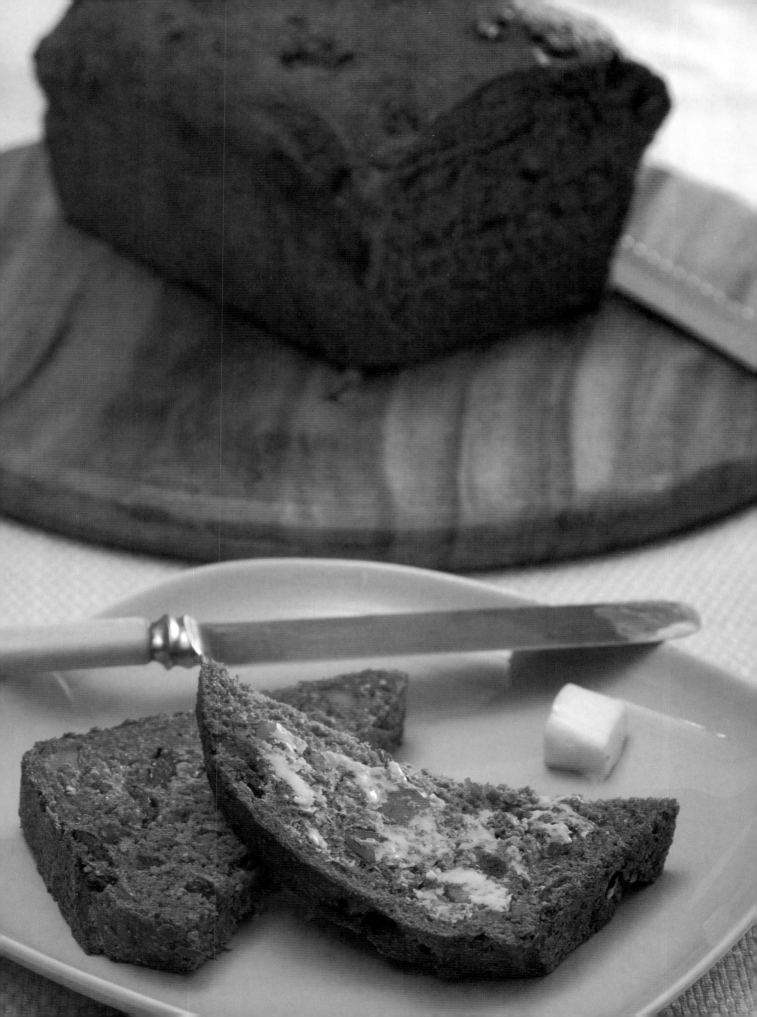

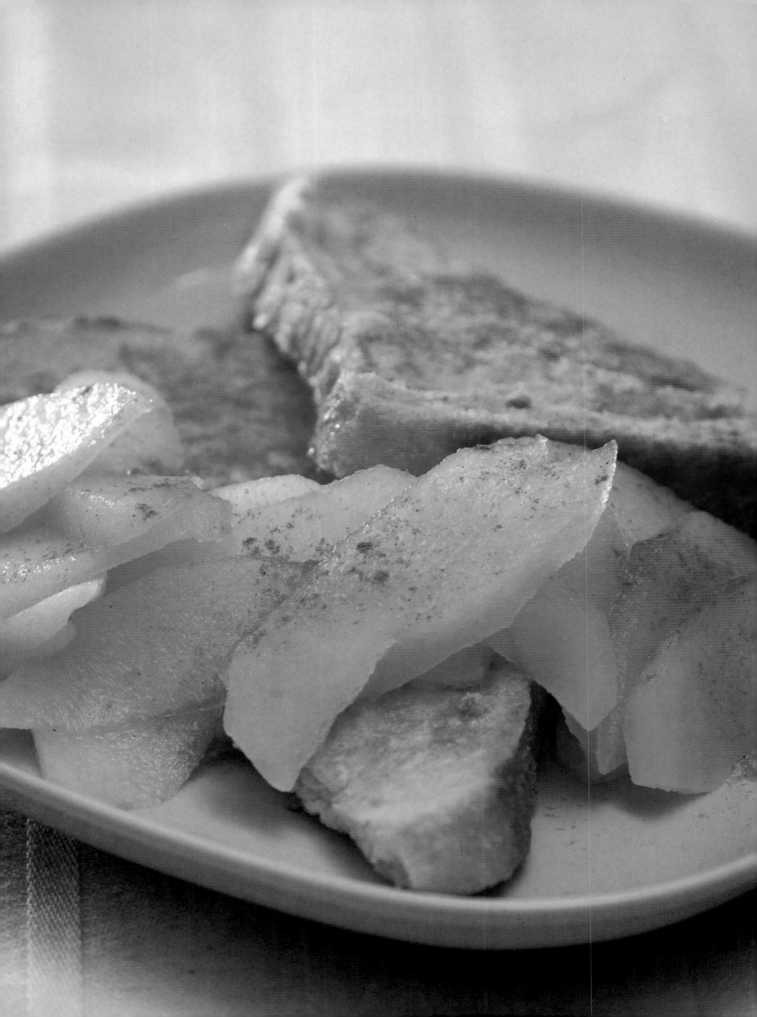

# Cinnamon Toast with Apple

*Family Favourite*

Protein from the eggs, carbohydrate from the bread, plus one portion of your daily five fruit and vegetables, this is a breakfast that should see you through to lunchtime.

## Serves 2

**2 large eating apples**
**2 large eggs**
**75ml/2½fl oz semi-skimmed milk**
**½ tsp vanilla essence**
**2 thick slices wholemeal bread**
**2 tsp brown sugar**
**pinch cinnamon**
**Greek yoghurt to serve**

## Serves 4

**4 large eating apples**
**4 large eggs**
**150ml/¼pt semi-skimmed milk**
**1 tsp vanilla essence**
**4 thick slices wholemeal bread**
**4 tsp brown sugar**
**large pinch cinnamon**
**Greek yoghurt to serve**

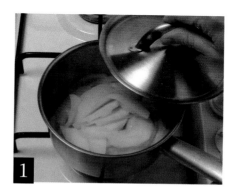

1 Peel and thinly slice the apples and place in a small pan with 4 (8) tbsp cold water. Bring gently to the boil. Cover and simmer for approximately 10 minutes until the apples are tender. Remove from the heat and keep warm while you prepare the bread.

2 Beat the eggs, milk and vanilla essence together in a shallow container large enough to take a slice of the bread. Dip 1 slice of the bread into the egg mixture, turning it to coat. Leave the bread in the egg mixture for 1–2 minutes so it can soak some of it up.

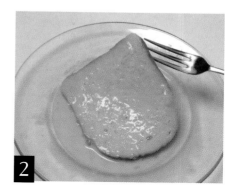

3 Heat a non-stick frying pan over a moderate heat and then cook the soaked bread for 3–4 minutes, turning halfway through, until golden and firm. Remove from the pan and keep warm while you repeat the method with the remaining slices.

4 To serve, place one slice of the cooked bread on each plate, sprinkle with a teaspoon of brown sugar and a little cinnamon. Top with the cooked apples and a spoonful of Greek yoghurt. Serve.

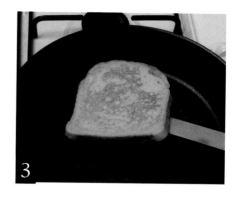

# Banana & Walnut Muffins

*Children's Choice*

Wholemeal flour, walnuts and bananas are healthy additions to these quick-and-easy muffins.

### Makes 10

**175g/6oz self-raising flour**
**100g/4oz wholemeal flour**
**1 tsp baking powder**
**1 tsp mixed spice**
**100g/4oz soft brown sugar**
**3 tbsp sunflower oil**
**2 large eggs**
**175ml/6fl oz semi-skimmed milk**
**2 ripe bananas**
**100g/4oz chopped walnuts**

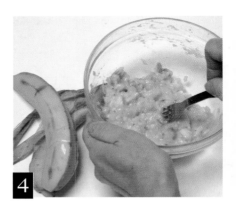

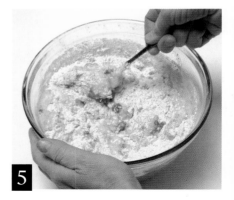

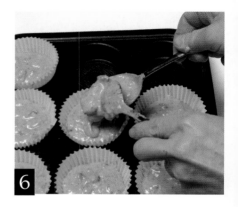

1 Preheat the oven to 190°C/375°F/Gas Mark 5. Line a muffin pan with 10 paper cases.

2 Sift the flours, baking powder and mixed spice together into a mixing bowl. Stir in the sugar. Make a well in the centre and set to one side until ready to use.

3 Beat the sunflower oil and eggs together. Add the milk and beat again.

4 Mash the banana and add to the egg and milk mixture, stirring.

5 Pour the banana mixture into the well, add the walnuts and stir quickly to combine. It is best not to overmix.

6 Divide the batter between the paper cases. Bake in the preheated oven for 25–30 minutes or until golden and risen. Cool on a wire rack for 5 minutes. Best served warm.

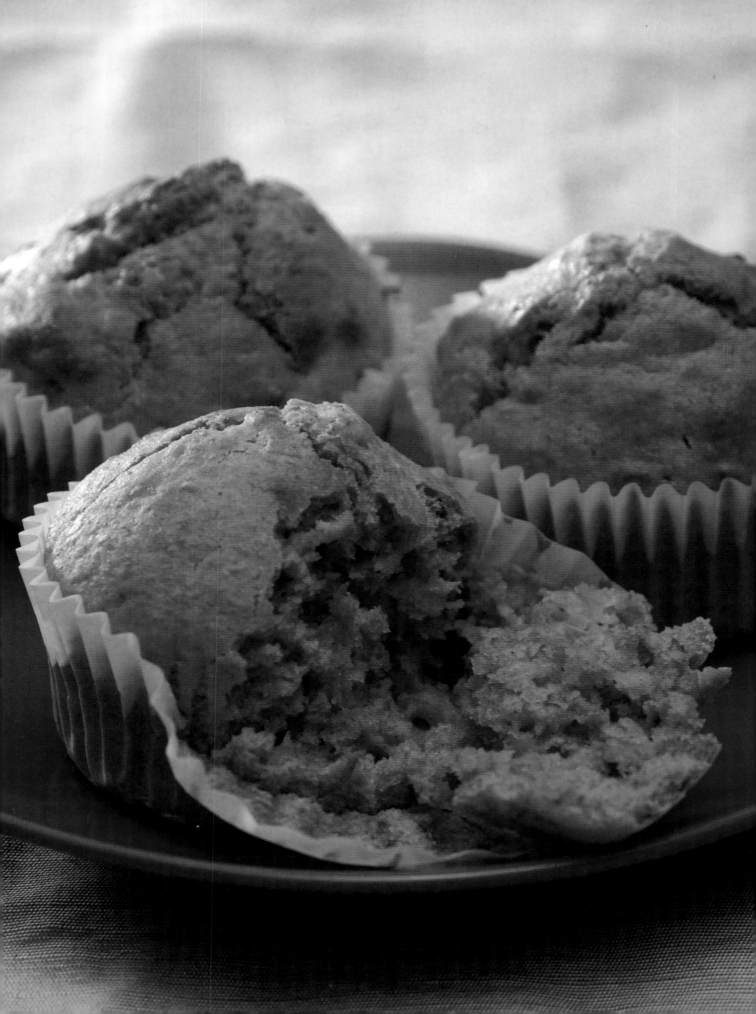

# Drop Scones & Berries

### Easy Entertaining

The choice of berries is up to you, but blueberries and strawberries are packed with the antioxidant vitamin C, vital for a healthy diet.

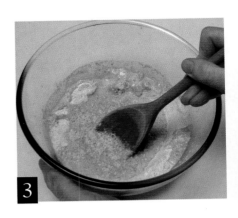

### Serves 2

**50g/2oz wholemeal flour**
**¼ tsp bicarbonate of soda**
**¼ tsp cream of tartar**
**1 tbsp honey**
**½ egg, beaten**
**75ml/2½fl oz semi-skimmed milk**
**50g/2oz blueberries**
**50g/2oz raspberries and/or strawberries**

### Serves 4

**100g/4oz wholemeal flour**
**½ tsp bicarbonate of soda**
**½ tsp cream of tartar**
**2 tbsp honey**
**1 egg, beaten**
**150ml/¼pt semi-skimmed milk**
**100g/4oz blueberries**
**100g/4oz raspberries and/or strawberries**

1 Place the flour in a mixing bowl and add the bicarbonate of soda and cream of tartar, ensuring there are no lumps. Stir well to mix, then form a well.

2 Beat the honey and egg together, then add the milk and beat again. Pour this mixture into the well.

3 Using a wooden spoon stir the milk mixture, drawing the flour in as you do so. Keep doing this until all the flour has been incorporated and the mixture is smooth. Beat well then set to one side.

4 Place about a third of the berries in a small saucepan with 1 (2) tbsp of cold water. Heat gently until the fruits are hot and their juices are starting to run. Stir in the remaining fruits and keep warm while you make the pancakes.

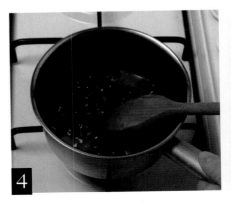

5 Heat a non-stick pan over a moderately high heat, then place tablespoons of the mixture into the pan and allow to cook undisturbed until small bubbles rise to the surface.

6 Turn each pancake and cook the other side until golden brown. Remove to a plate and keep warm while you cook the remainder. To serve, divide the pancakes between the plates and top with the warm berries.

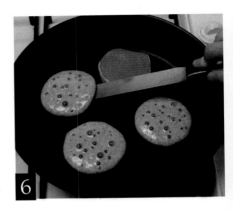

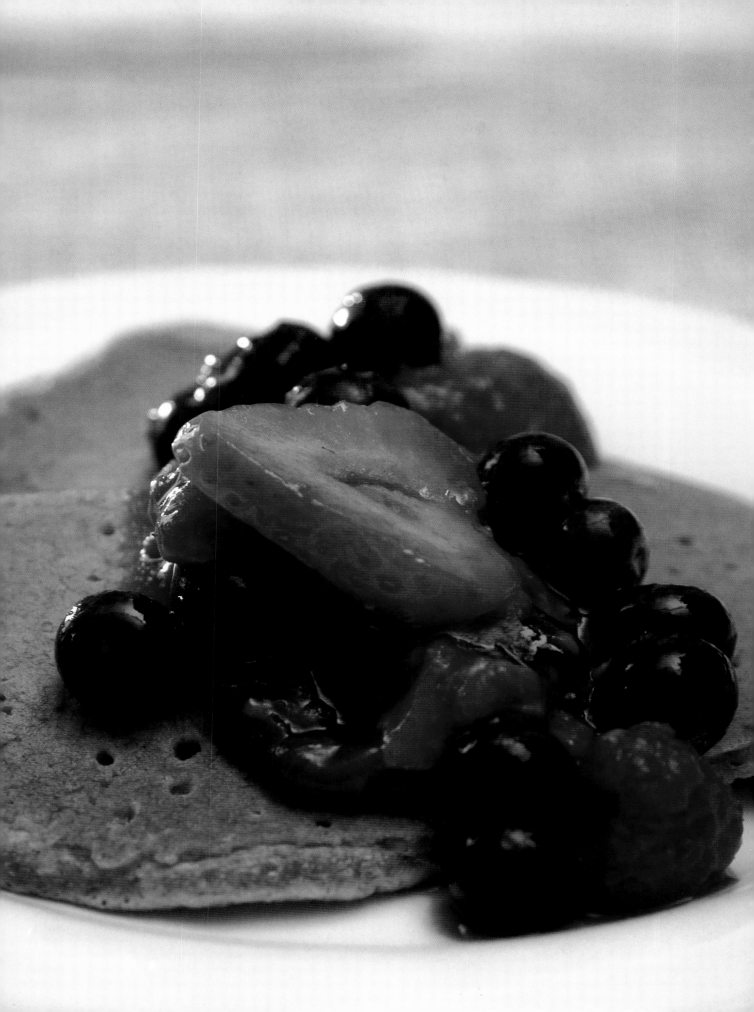

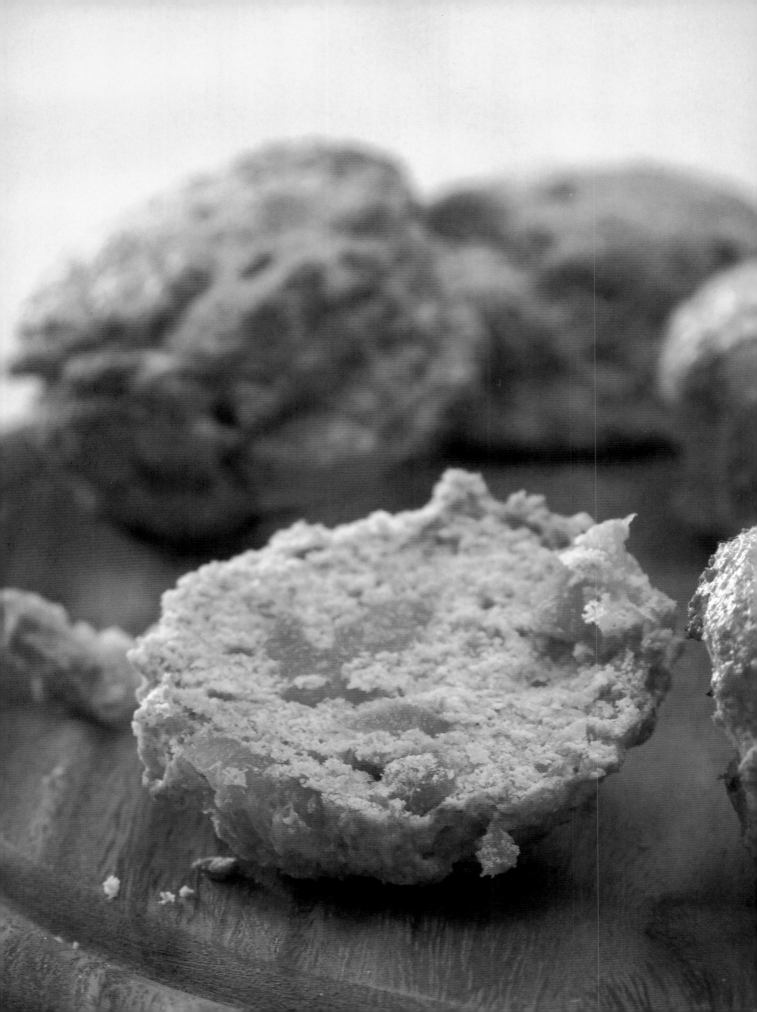

# Lemon & Apricot Scones

### *Children's Choice*

Dried apricots are not only high in fibre but also contain iron.

## Makes 8

**150g/ 5oz wholemeal self-raising flour**
**100g/4oz self-raising flour**
**25g/1oz butter**
**40g/1½oz soft brown sugar**
**125g/4½oz dried ready-to-eat apricots**
**1 unwaxed lemon**
**1 egg**
**4 tbsp milk**

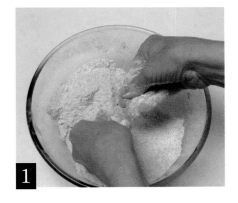

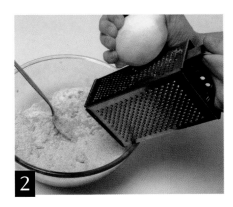

1 Preheat the oven to 220°C/425°F/Gas Mark 7. Mix the flours together in a mixing bowl. Cut the butter into small pieces, add to the flour and rub in.

2 Stir in the sugar. Finely chop the apricots and stir through the flour mixture. Finely grate the zest from the lemon and add to the mixture.

3 Beat the egg with the milk and add to this 2 tbsp of lemon juice from the zested lemon. Stir and then add this to the flour mixture, stirring to form a dough.

4 Turn out on to a lightly floured surface and roll out to a thickness of 2.5cm/1in. Cut out rounds with a 7.5cm/3in round cutter. Place on a lightly floured baking tray and cook in the preheated oven for 10–12 minutes until golden and risen. Cool on a wire rack for 5 minutes then serve warm.

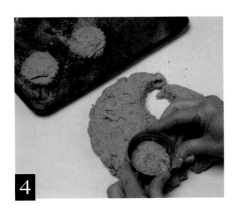

# Cranberry & Pecan Buns

*Family Favourite*

Wholesome buns, handy to have at the ready for lunch boxes or when you need a quick snack.

*Makes 8*

**175g/6oz wholemeal flour**
**1 tsp baking powder**
**75g/3oz butter or margarine**
**75g/3oz soft light brown sugar**
**100g/4oz dried cranberries**
**1 lemon**
**100g/4oz pecan nuts, roughly chopped**
**1 egg**

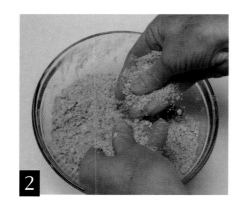

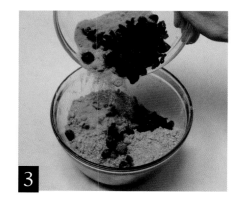

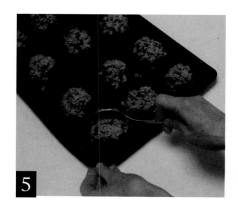

1 Preheat the oven to 220°C/425°F/Gas Mark 7. Lightly grease a large baking tray.

2 Place the flour and baking powder in a bowl and mix. Add the butter and cut into pieces. Now rub in the butter until the mixture resembles coarse breadcrumbs.

3 Stir in the sugar and cranberries. Finely grate the zest from the lemon and add, stirring well to mix.

4 Stir in the chopped pecans. Beat the egg and add to the mixture along with enough lemon juice to make a stiff dough.

5 Place heaped spoonfuls on the prepared baking tray, leaving space between each one to allow for rising. Bake in the preheated oven for 15 minutes until golden and risen. Cool on a wire rack before storing in an airtight container.

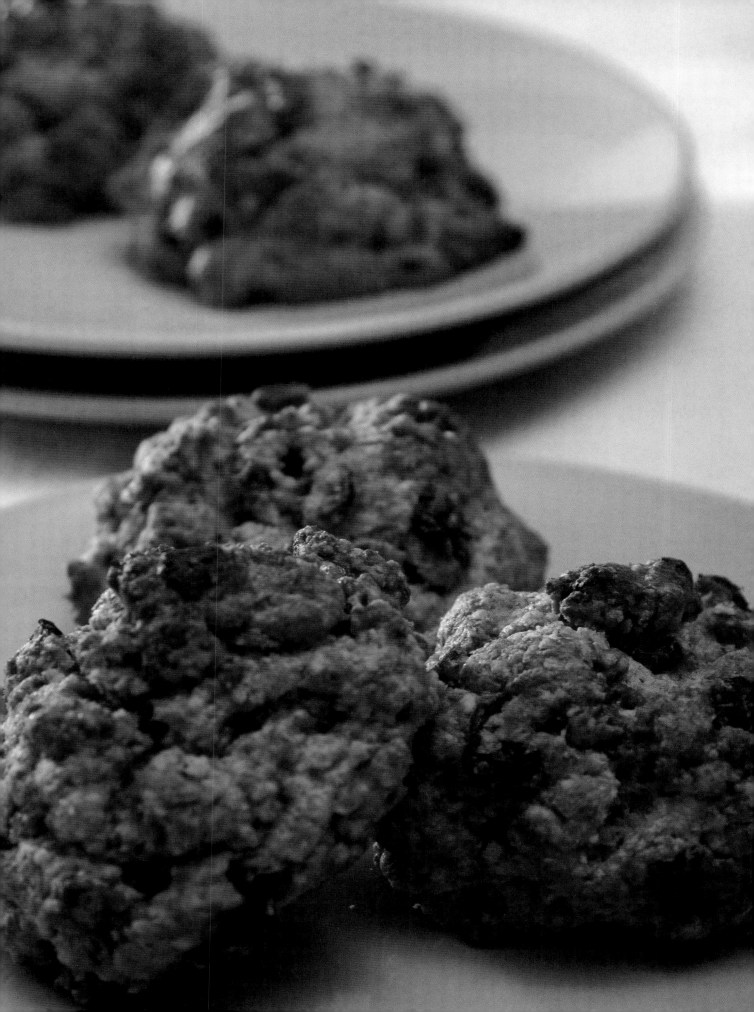

# Flapjacks

*Family Favourite*

Crumbly flapjacks full of juicy apricots make a great snack to keep you going. Rolled oats are a slow-burn carbohydrate and apricots are an excellent source of iron.

*Makes 9*

**100g/4oz ready-to-eat dried apricots**
**2 pieces of preserved stem ginger**
**100g/4oz butter**
**4 tbsp honey**
**3 tbsp demerara sugar**
**150g/5oz rolled oats**
**25g/1oz sesame seeds**
**1 heaped tbsp wholemeal flour**

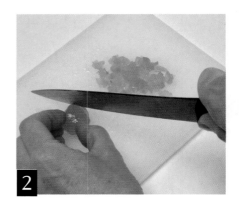

1 Preheat the oven to 190°C/375°F/Gas Mark 5. Grease and base line an 18cm/7in square tin.

2 Chop the apricots and set to one side. Finely chop the stem ginger, add to the chopped apricots and mix.

3 Place the butter, honey and sugar in a pan over a moderate heat, stirring from time to time until they are melted and fully mixed.

4 Remove the pan from the heat and stir in the oats, sesame seeds and flour, mixing well to coat in honey mixture.

5 Add the apricots and ginger and mix again. Press the mixture into the prepared tin and bake in the preheated oven for 25 minutes.

6 Remove from the oven and place the tin on a wire cooling rack. Mark into squares using a sharp knife, then leave to cool fully before removing from the tin. Store in an airtight container.

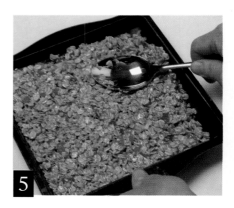

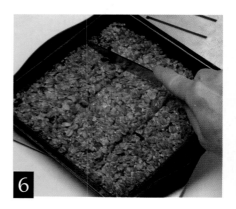

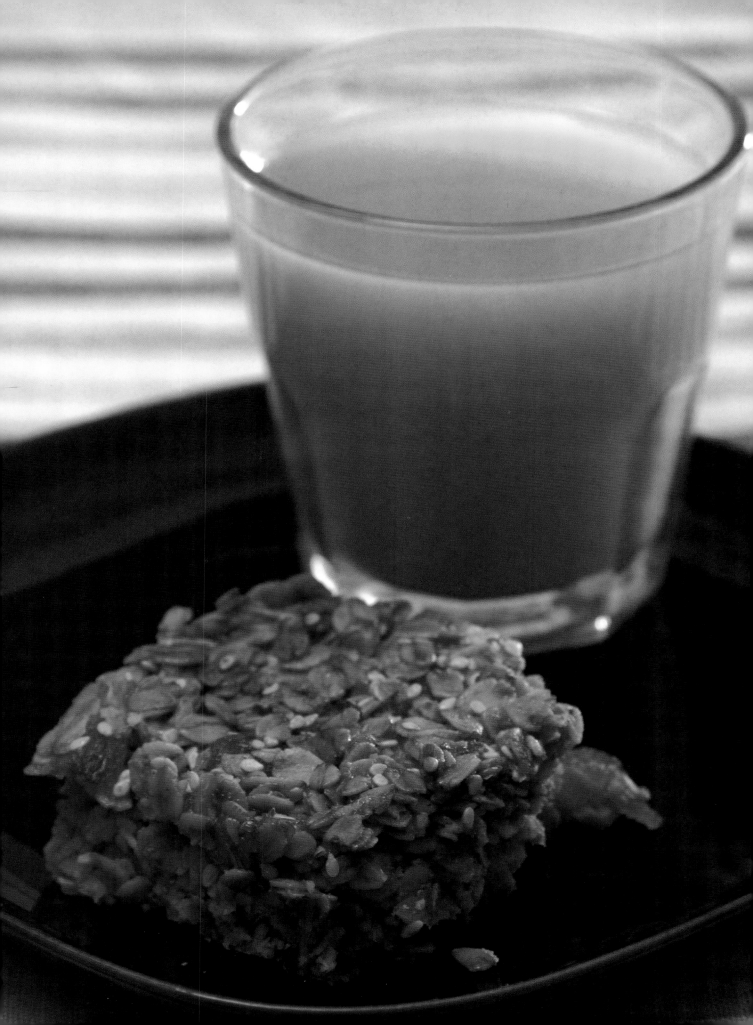

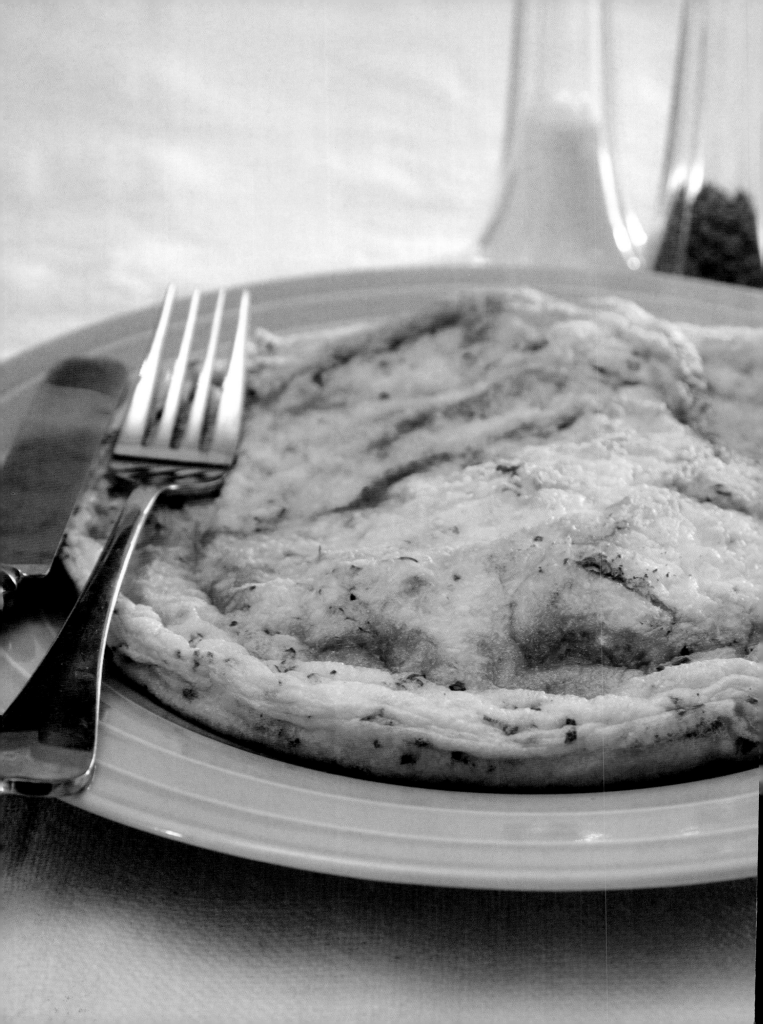

# Herb Omelette

*vegetarian*

If you wish to make one large omelette, use a big frying pan and slice the omelette after cooking. If you prefer, vegetarian Parmesan is now widely available from supermarkets and specialist shops.

## Serves 2

**4 eggs**
**2 tbsp parsley chopped**
**1 tbsp chives chopped**
**butter for greasing**
**15g/½oz Parmesan, finely**
 **grated**
**salt and freshly ground**
 **black pepper to taste**

## Serves 4

**8 eggs**
**4 tbsp parsley chopped**
**2 tbsp chives chopped**
**butter for greasing**
**25g/1oz Parmesan, finely**
 **grated**
**salt and freshly ground**
 **black pepper to taste**

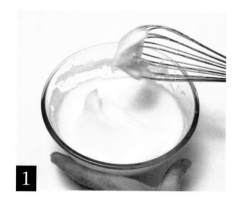

1 Separate the eggs and beat the yolks together with a little salt and pepper. Now, using a whisk, whip the egg whites until they reach soft-peak stage.

2 Using a large metal spoon, gently fold the egg whites and chopped herbs into the egg yolks. Preheat the grill to high.

3 Lightly grease a small frying pan with a little butter and place over a moderate heat. Add half (a quarter) of the egg mixture and cook for 2–3 minutes. Scatter over half (a quarter) of the Parmesan, then place the pan under the preheated grill. Cook for 1 minute until golden in places and springy to the touch. Remove from the heat and serve. Repeat with the remaining mixture.

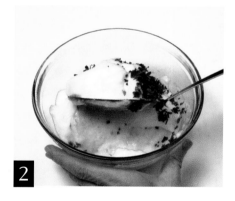

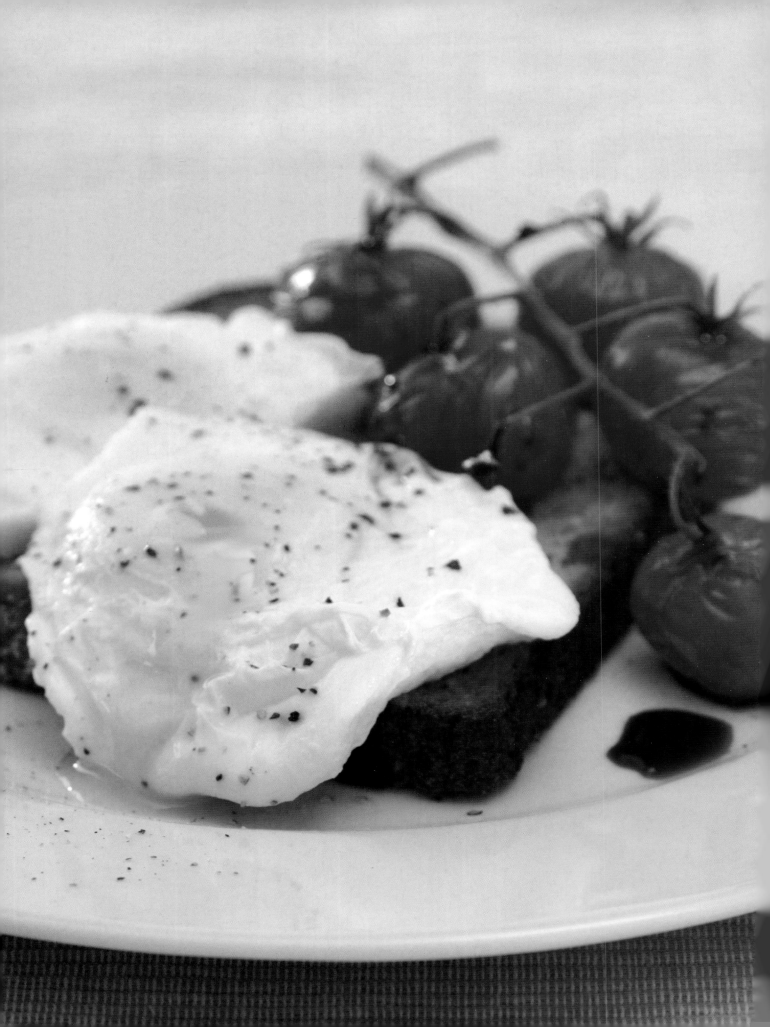

# Grilled Cherry Tomatoes with Poached Eggs

*Quick and Easy*

Eggs are high in cholesterol but they have so much more in their favour – just eat them in moderation. They are an excellent source of vitamin B12, rich in vitamins and minerals and a good source of protein

### Serves 2

**175g/6oz cherry tomatoes**
**4 eggs**
**2 thick slices wholemeal**
    **bread**
**2 tsp balsamic vinegar**
**freshly ground black pepper**

### Serves 4

**350g/12oz cherry tomatoes**
**8 eggs**
**4 thick slices wholemeal**
    **bread**
**4 tsp balsamic vinegar**
**freshly ground black pepper**

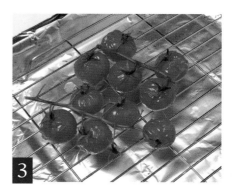

1 Preheat the grill to moderately high. Line the grill pan with foil.

2 Fill a frying pan with water and bring to the boil.

3 Wash the tomatoes and arrange them in a single layer in the grill pan. Cook them under the preheated grill for 5–8 minutes until they start to lose their shape a little and their skins wrinkle.

4 While the tomatoes are cooking, and when the water has boiled, carefully break one egg into a cup and then slide the egg into the boiling water.

5 Repeat with the remaining eggs. Cook the eggs for 3 minutes, basting them with the boiling water if their tops are showing above the water.

6 Toast the bread and place a slice on each plate. Divide the eggs and tomatoes between the plates, drizzle with the balsamic vinegar and season with freshly ground black pepper. Serve.

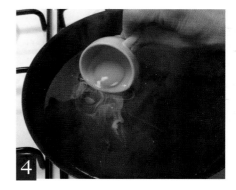

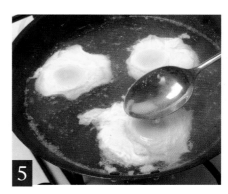

# Parma Ham & Scrambled Eggs

*Family Favourite*

I find Parma ham a fantastic alternative for when I am having a real bacon craving.

## Serves 2

**3 eggs**
**1 tbsp semi-skimmed milk**
**4 slices Parma ham**
**a small knob of butter**
**2 slices of wholemeal bread**
**freshly ground black pepper**

## Serves 4

**6 eggs**
**2 tbsp semi-skimmed milk**
**8 slices Parma ham**
**a knob of butter**
**4 slices whole meal bread.**
**freshly ground black pepper**

1 Preheat the grill. Beat the eggs and milk together.

2 Cook the Parma ham for 1–2 minutes under the preheated grill, turning halfway through. Remove and keep warm while you cook the eggs.

3 Melt the butter in a small, preferably non-stick, pan. Add the beaten eggs and cook, stirring all the time, over a moderate heat until the eggs are set and firm.

4 Toast the bread. Place a slice on each plate. Divide the eggs between the slices of toast. Season with black pepper and top with the grilled Parma ham. Serve.

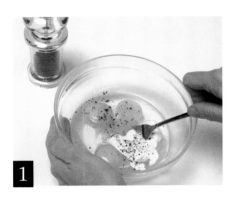

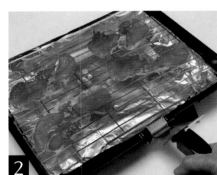

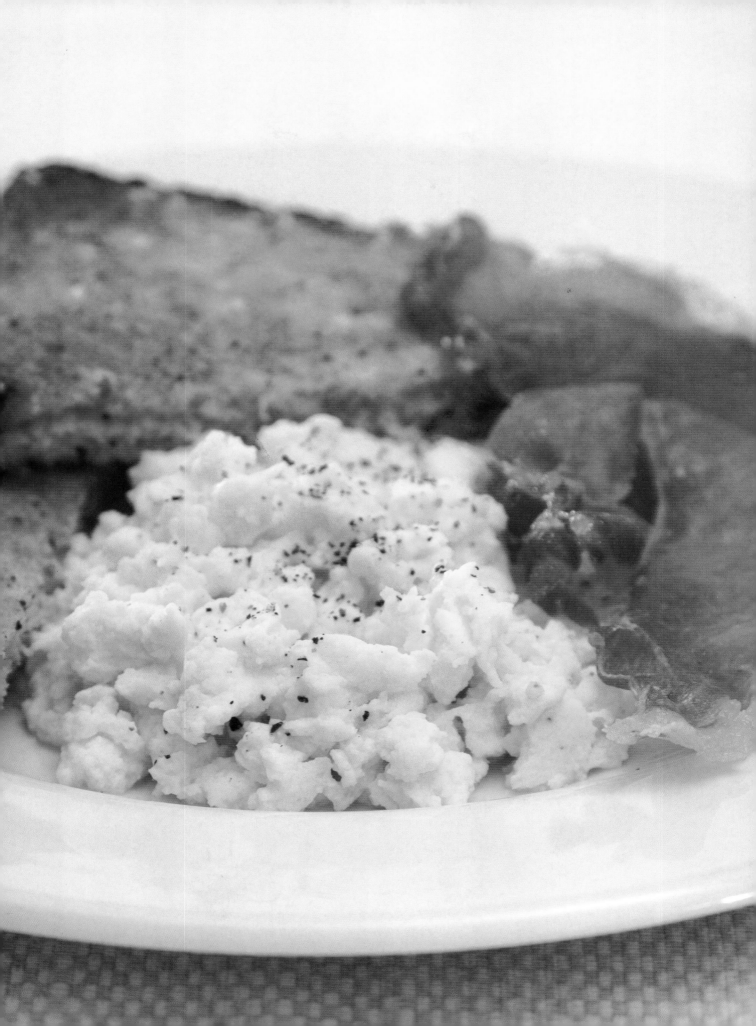

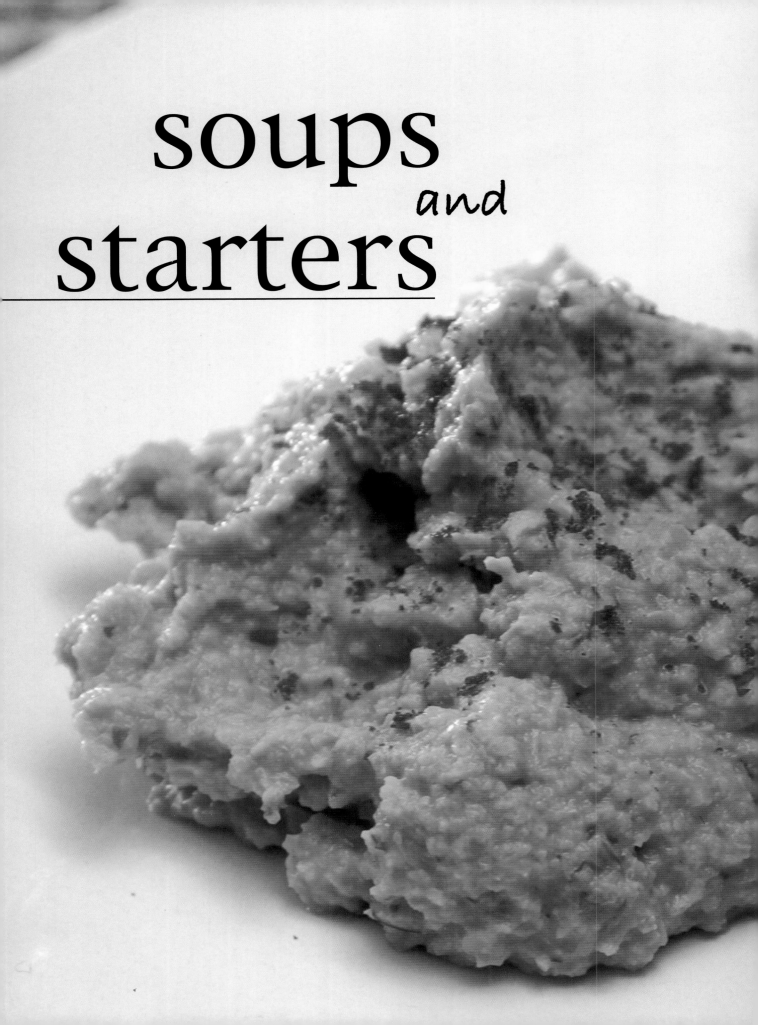

# soups and starters

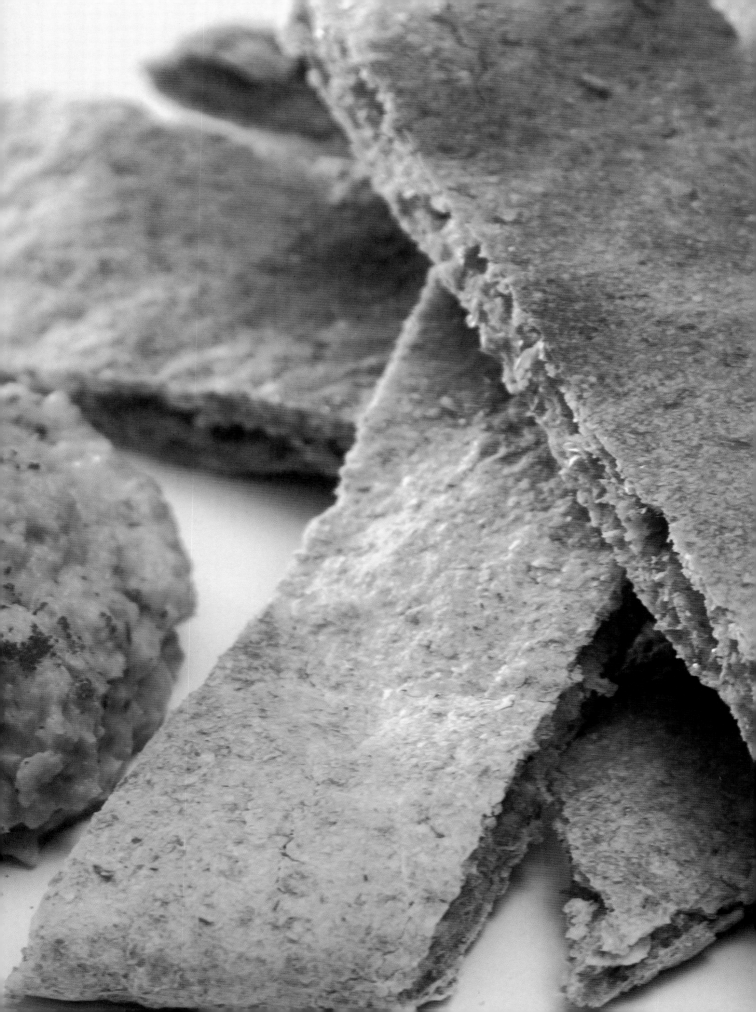

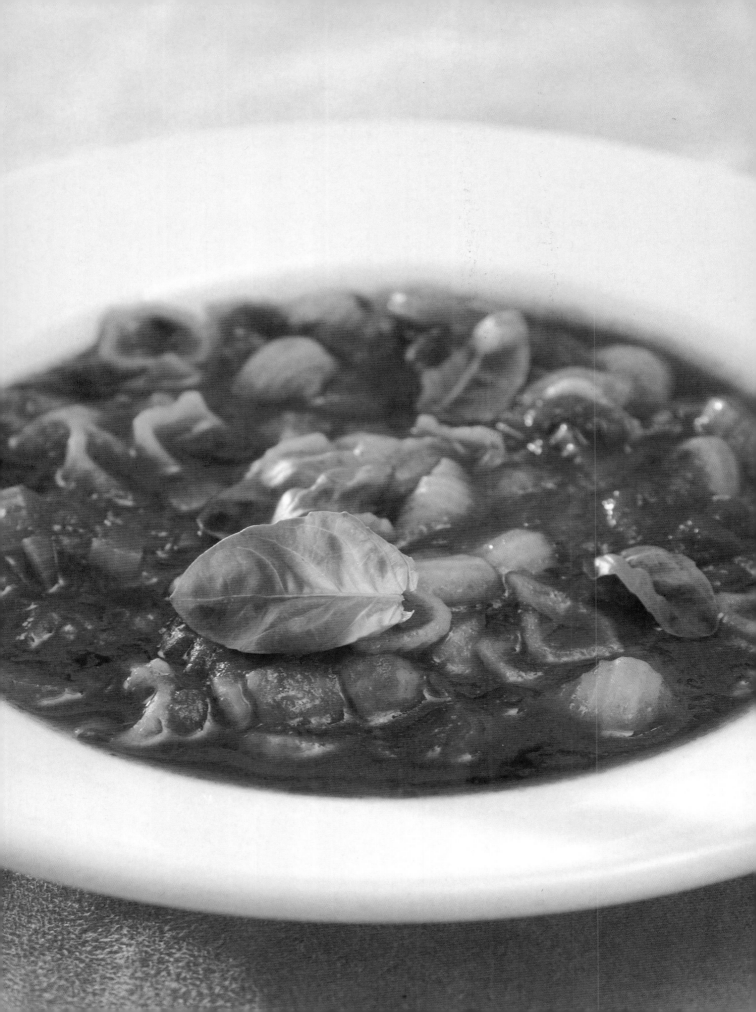

# Tomato Soup

## Children's Choice

Soup is a tasty, healthy lunch. The addition of pasta gives some of the carbohydrate needed to keep you going until the next mealtime.

### Serves 2

1 tbsp olive oil
1 clove garlic, peeled and crushed
1 small onion, peeled and finely chopped
2 sticks celery, chopped
1 x 400g/14oz can tomatoes, chopped
2 tbsp fresh basil, chopped
50g/2oz small pasta
salt and freshly ground black pepper
basil leaves to garnish

### Serves 4

2 tbsp olive oil
2 cloves garlic, peeled and crushed
1 onion, peeled and finely chopped
4 sticks celery, chopped
2 x 400g/14oz cans tomatoes, chopped
4 tbsp fresh basil, chopped
100g/4oz small pasta
salt and freshly ground black pepper
basil leaves to garnish

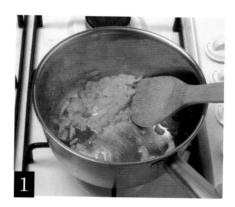

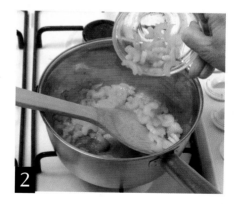

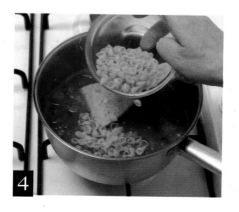

1 Heat the oil in a large saucepan. Add the garlic and onion and cook over a gentle heat until the onion is softened and transparent.

2 Add the celery and cook for a further 3–4 minutes, stirring from time to time.

3 Add the tomatoes and basil and stir. Pour over 300ml/½pt (600ml/1pt) of water and increase the heat to bring to the boil.

4 Add the pasta and reduce the heat to a gentle simmer. Cook, covered, for 15 minutes. Remove from the heat, season to taste and serve garnished with basil leaves.

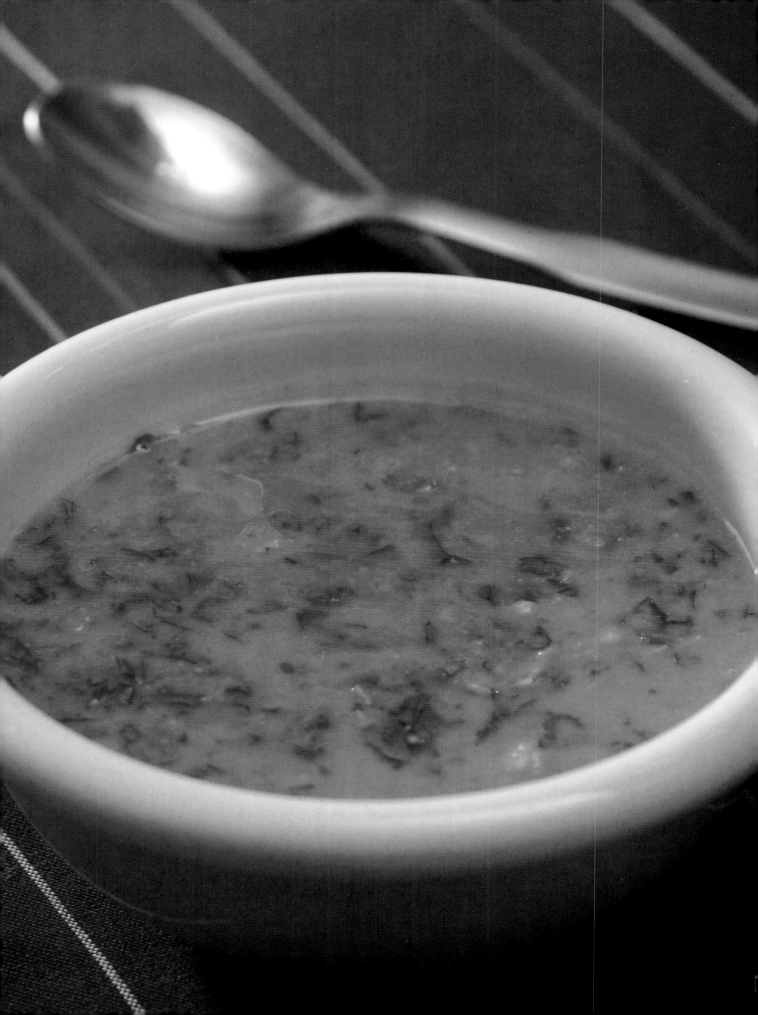

# Chickpea Soup

*vegetarian*

Pulses are low in fat and help lower cholesterol. They are also a good supply of protein and fibre.

## Serves 2

**1 red onion, peeled**
**1 tbsp olive oil**
**1 x 200g/7oz can chickpeas**
**600ml/1pt vegetable stock**
**2 tbsp fresh parsley,**
    **chopped**
**2 tbsp fresh mint, chopped**
**2 tbsp fresh coriander,**
    **chopped**
**salt and freshly ground**
    **black pepper**

## Serves 4

**1 large red onion, peeled**
**2 tbsp olive oil**
**1 x 400g/14oz can chickpeas**
**1.2l/2pt vegetable stock**
**4 tbsp fresh parsley,**
    **chopped**
**4 tbsp fresh mint, chopped**
**4 tbsp fresh coriander,**
    **chopped**
**salt and freshly ground**
    **black pepper**

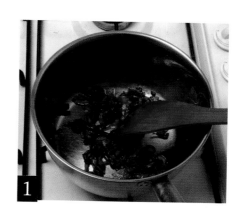

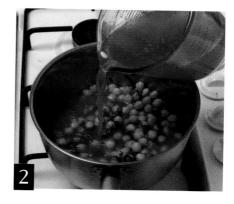

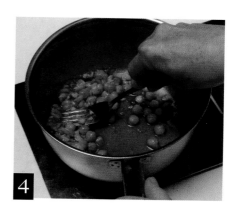

1 Halve the onion and slice it finely. Heat the oil in a large saucepan and cook the onion over a moderate heat until it softens. Reduce the heat and cook the onion gently until it starts to caramelise in places, stirring from time to time.

2 Drain the chickpeas and rinse well. Add to the onion and stir. Pour over the stock and bring to the boil.

3 Reduce the heat to a gentle simmer and cook, covered, for 15 minutes. Remove from the heat and allow the soup to cool for 10 minutes.

4 Pour ¾ of the soup into food processor or blender and process until smooth. Roughly mash the chickpeas in the remainder of the soup with a fork. If you prefer a completely smooth texture you can blend all the soup.

5 Return all the soup to the pan and gently reheat. Remove from the heat and stir in the freshly chopped herbs. Season to taste and serve.

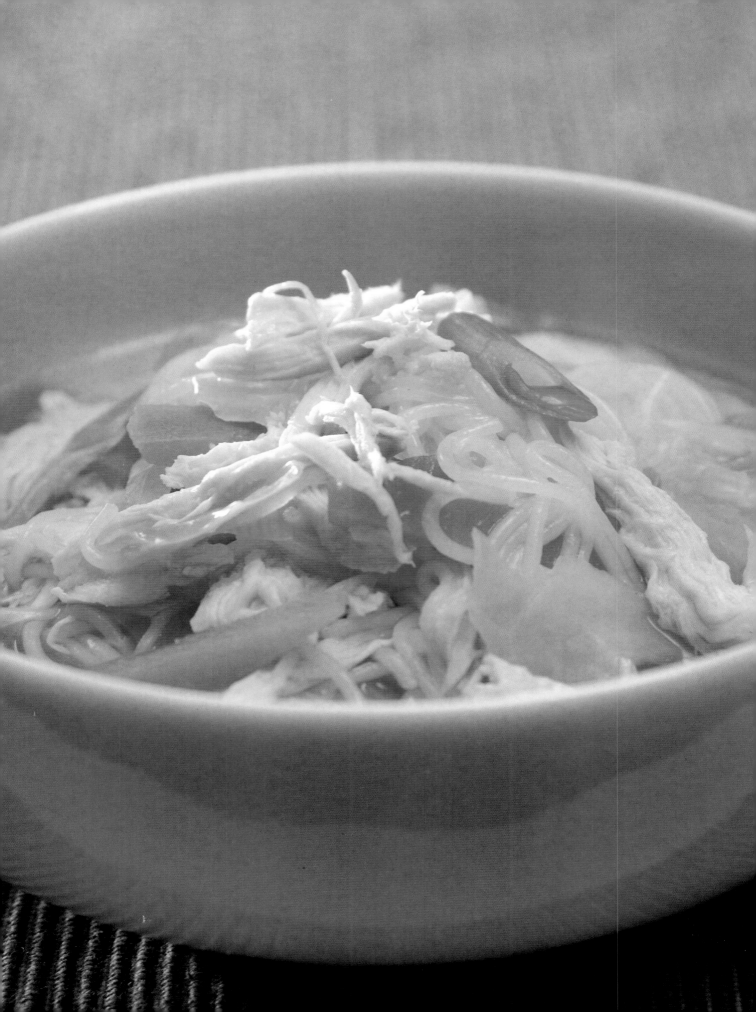

# Chicken Noodle Soup

*Family Favourite*

A delicious soup that is a meal in a bowl.

## Serves 2

**1 small stick lemon grass**
**2.5cm/1in fresh ginger, peeled and sliced**
**1 clove garlic, peeled and sliced**
**1 small onion, peeled and halved**
**4 black peppercorns**
**1 skinless chicken breast**
**½ chicken stock cube**
**1 large carrot, peeled and cut into matchsticks**
**4 spring onions, trimmed and sliced**
**100g/4oz green cabbage, shredded**
**50g/2oz rice vermicelli**

## Serves 4

**1 stick lemon grass**
**5cm/2in fresh ginger, peeled and sliced**
**2 cloves garlic, peeled and sliced**
**1 onion, peeled and halved**
**8 black peppercorns**
**2 skinless chicken breasts**
**1 chicken stock cube**
**2 large carrots, peeled and cut into matchsticks**
**8 spring onions, trimmed and sliced**
**200g/7oz green cabbage, shredded**
**100g/4oz rice vermicelli**

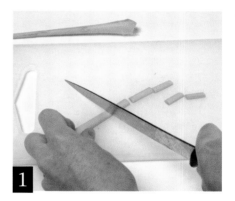

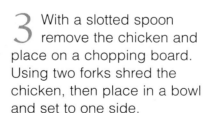

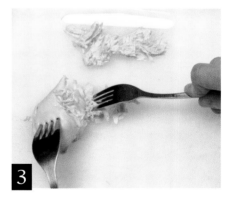

1 Remove the coarse outer layer from the lemon grass and discard. Cut the lemon grass into 2.5cm/1in lengths.

2 Place the lemon grass, ginger, garlic, onion, peppercorns and chicken breast in a large saucepan. Dissolve the stock cube in 450ml/¾pt (900ml/1½pt) boiling water. Pour into the saucepan and bring gently to the boil. Reduce the heat to a gentle simmer and cook, covered, for 15 minutes. Remove from the heat.

3 With a slotted spoon remove the chicken and place on a chopping board. Using two forks shred the chicken, then place in a bowl and set to one side.

4 Strain the stock from the pan and discard the lemon grass, ginger, etc.

5 Return the stock to the pan and bring to the boil. Add the carrots, spring onions, cabbage and vermicelli and cook for 4–5 minutes. Stir in the shredded chicken and cook for a further 1–2 minutes. Serve.

# Curried Lentil Soup

## *vegetarian*

Lentils are a good source of fibre and protein.

### Serves 2

**2 tsp olive oil**
**1 clove garlic, peeled and crushed**
**1 small onion, peeled and finely chopped**
**1 stick celery, finely chopped**
**½ tbsp curry powder**
**50g/2oz red lentils, rinsed and drained**
**1 x 100g/4oz can tomatoes, chopped**
**½ vegetable stock cube**
**2 tbsp fresh coriander, chopped**
**1 tbsp plain yoghurt**

### Serves 4

**4 tsp olive oil**
**2 cloves garlic, peeled and crushed**
**1 onion, peeled and finely chopped**
**2 sticks celery, finely chopped**
**1 tbsp curry powder**
**100g/4oz red lentils, rinsed and drained**
**1 x 200g/7oz can tomatoes, chopped**
**1 vegetable stock cube**
**4 tbsp fresh coriander, chopped**
**2 tbsp plain yoghurt**

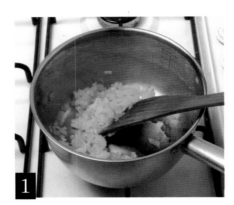

1 Heat the oil in a large saucepan over a moderate heat. Add the garlic, onion and celery and cook, stirring from time to time, until softened.

2 Add the curry powder and cook, stirring for 1–2 minutes. Add the lentils and stir well to coat them in the spiced onion mixture.

3 Stir in the chopped tomatoes. Dissolve the stock cube in 450ml/¾pt (750ml/1¼pt) boiling water. Add this to the pan and bring to the boil. Reduce the heat to a gentle simmer and cook, covered, for 15 minutes until the lentils are tender.

4 Remove from the heat and stir through the chopped coriander. Serve topped with a spoonful of yoghurt in each bowl.

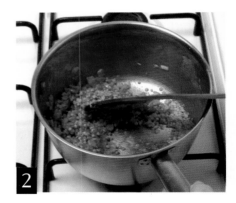

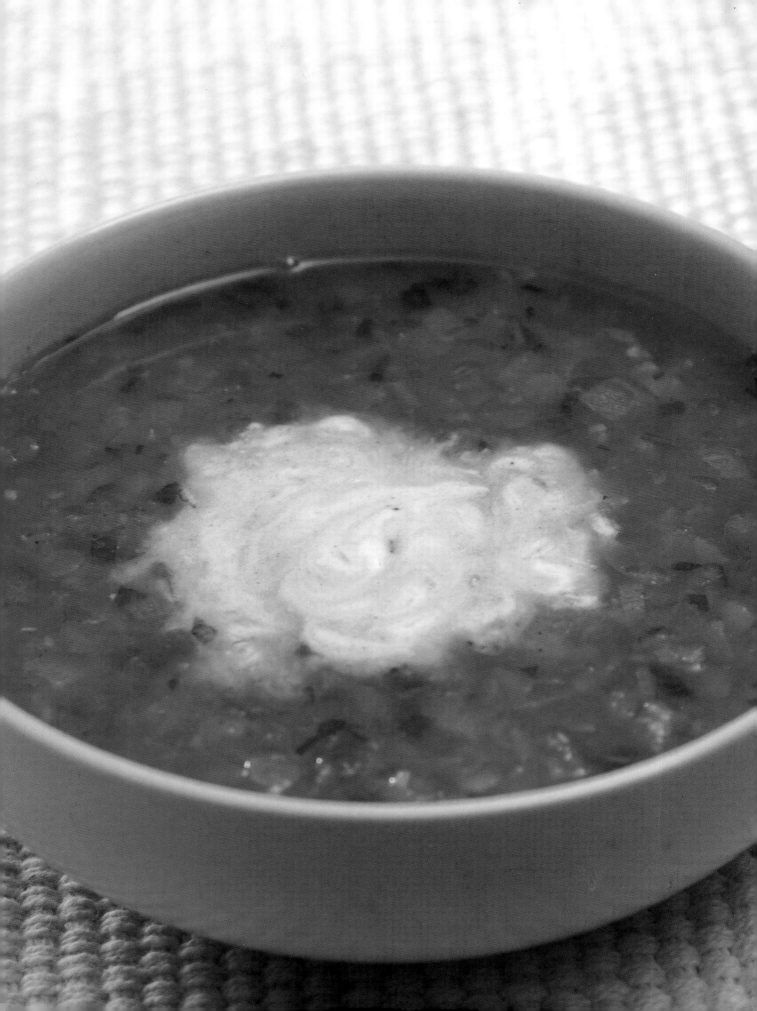

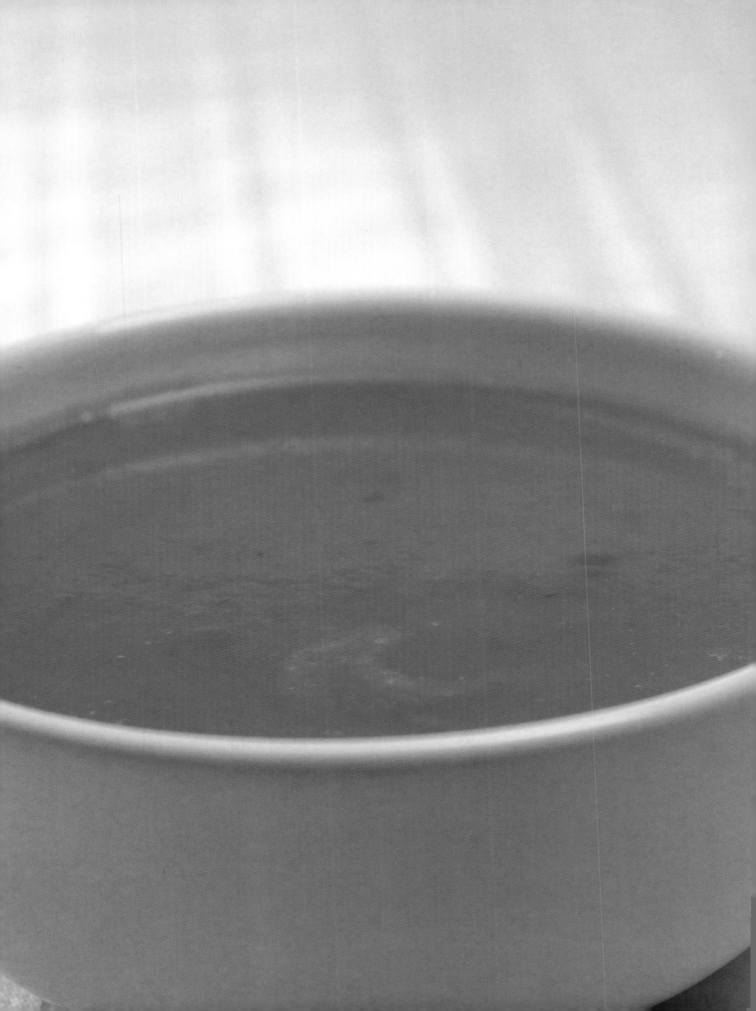

# Carrot & Thyme Soup

*Family Favourite*

Homemade soups are so easy you will wonder why you ever considered buying them instead.

### Serves 2

**1 tbsp olive oil**
**1 small onion, peeled and chopped**
**1 clove garlic, peeled and crushed**
**450g/1lb carrots, peeled and chopped**
**1 chicken stock cube**
**1 tbsp yeast extract**
**½ tsp dried thyme**

### Serves 4

**2 tbsp olive oil**
**1 onion, peeled and chopped**
**2 cloves garlic, peeled and crushed**
**900g/2lb carrots, peeled and chopped**
**2 chicken stock cubes**
**2 tbsp yeast extract**
**1 tsp dried thyme**

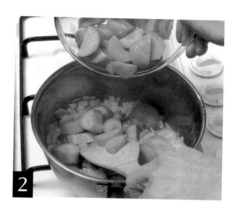

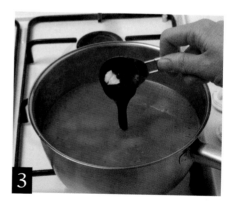

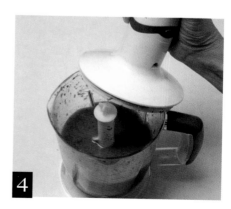

1 Heat the oil in a large saucepan and cook the onion and garlic over a moderate heat until softened.

2 Add the carrots and stir well. Cover with a well-fitting lid and reduce the heat to low. Cook for 15 minutes shaking the pan from time to time to mix.

3 Dissolve the stock cubes in 600ml/1pt (1.2l/2pt) of boiling water. Add this to the pan along with the yeast extract and dried thyme. Bring to the boil, then reduce the heat to a gentle simmer.

4 Replace the lid and cook, covered, for 20 minutes. Remove from the heat and allow the soup to cool for 10 minutes. Using a food processor or blender, process the soup until it is smooth and return it to the pan. Gently reheat until it is piping hot and serve.

# Roasted Vegetable & Rice Soup

*vegetarian*

By making soup yourself you ensure that all the ingredients are fresh and, of course, the cost is at least half what it would be if it was ready made.

## Serves 2

**50g/2oz brown rice**
**1 small carrot**
**1 small parsnip**
**1 tbsp olive oil**
**1 small red pepper**
**1 small courgette**
**2 garlic cloves**
**600ml/1pt vegetable stock**

## Serves 4

**100g/4oz brown rice**
**1 large carrot**
**1 large parsnip**
**2 tbsp olive oil**
**1 large red pepper**
**1 large courgette**
**4 garlic cloves**
**1.2l/2pt vegetable stock**

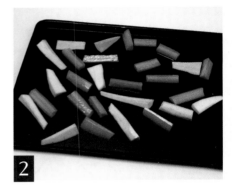

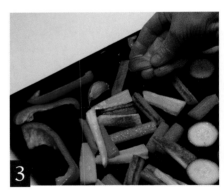

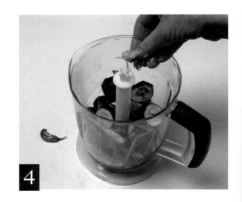

1 Cook the brown rice according to the pack instructions, then drain and set to one side. Preheat the oven to 200°C/400°F/Gas Mark 6. Line a baking tray with parchment paper.

2 Peel and cut the carrot and parsnip into large batons. Place in a mixing bowl and drizzle over the olive oil. Toss well to coat, then spread in a single layer over the prepared baking tray and cook for 15 minutes.

3 Deseed the pepper and cut into strips. Trim the courgette and cut into chunks.

Toss the courgette and pepper into the parsnip and carrot. Add the unpeeled cloves of garlic and cook for a further 15 minutes.

4 When cool enough to handle, squeeze the cooked garlic from their skins and discard the skins. Add the cooked flesh to the vegetables and then process in a food processor or blender until roughly chopped.

5 Now place this mixture in a large saucepan, adding the stock and cooked rice. Bring to the boil and cook, covered, for 10 minutes. Serve.

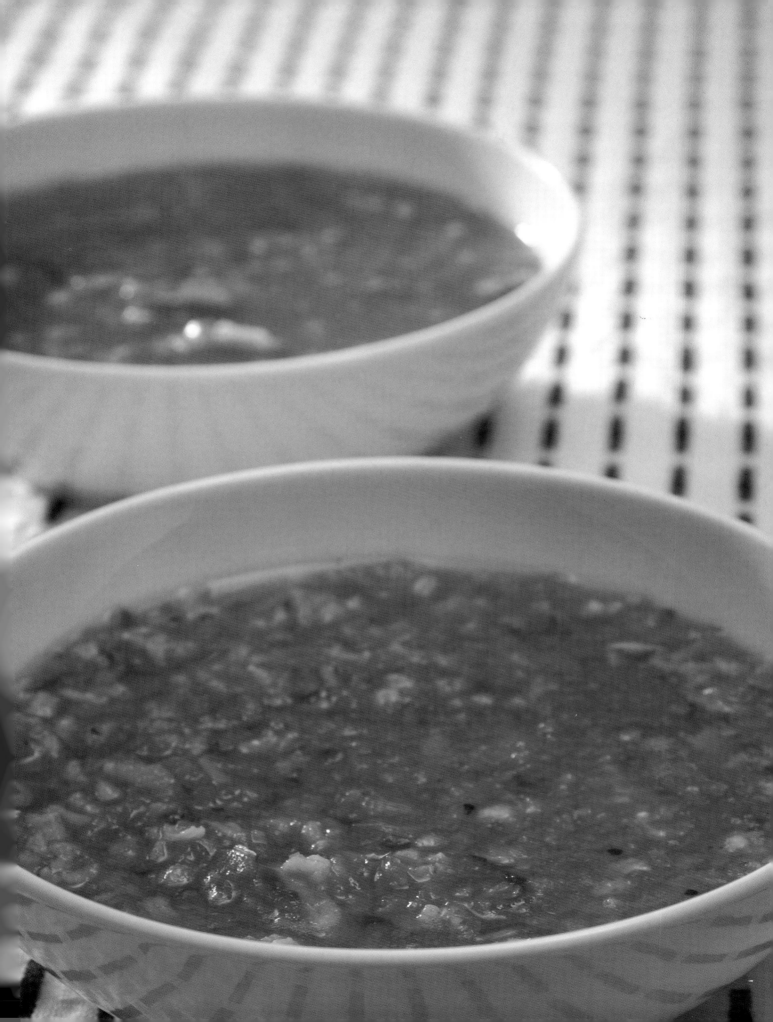

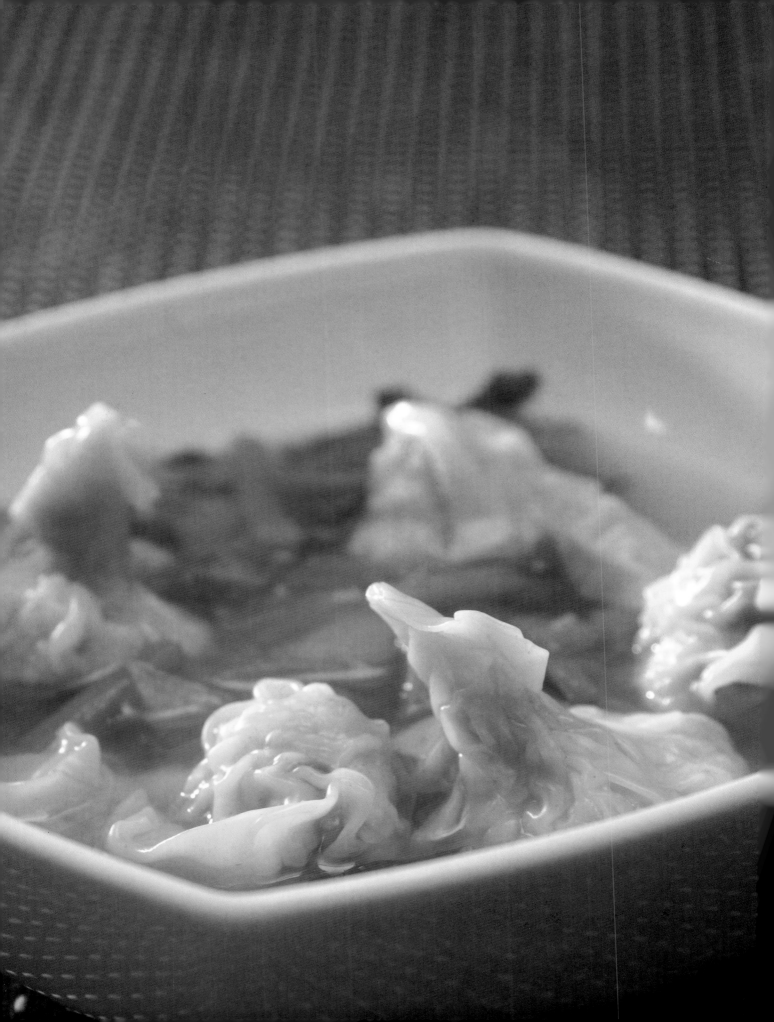

# Won Ton Soup with Pak Choi

*Easy Entertaining*

A low-fat soup that is full of flavour.

## Serves 2

4 spring onions
4 shitake mushrooms
100g/4oz chicken breast
¼ tsp sesame oil
1cm/½in fresh ginger,
    peeled and finely grated
1 small clove garlic, peeled
    and crushed
pinch chilli powder
10 fresh won ton wrappers
600ml/1pt chicken stock
1 large carrot, peeled and cut
    into matchsticks
2 pak choi, shredded

## Serves 4

8 spring onions
8 shitake mushrooms
200g/7oz chicken breast
½ tsp sesame oil
2.5cm/1in fresh ginger,
    peeled and finely grated
1 clove garlic, peeled and
    crushed
¼ tsp chilli powder
20 fresh won ton wrappers
1.2l/2pt chicken stock
2 large carrots, peeled and
    cut into matchsticks
4 pak choi, shredded

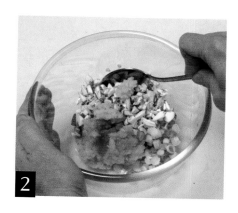

1 Trim and finely shred the spring onions. Clean and finely chop the shitake mushrooms.

2 Place the chicken in a food processor or blender and chop finely. Place the spring onions, mushrooms, chicken, sesame oil, grated ginger, garlic and chilli powder in a bowl and mix well.

3 Brush the edges of a won ton wrapper with a little cold water, then take a heaped teaspoon of the chicken mixture and place it in the middle of the wrapper.

4 Draw the edges of wrapper up tightly around the filling. Pinch the edges together to seal and set to one side while you repeat the procedure with the remaining filling and wrappers.

5 Place the chicken stock in a large saucepan and bring to the boil. Add the carrots and won tons and cook, covered, for 5 minutes. Roughly slice the pak choi and then add to the pan and cook for a further 2–3 minutes until tender. Remove from the heat and serve.

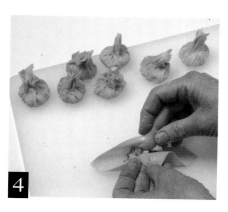

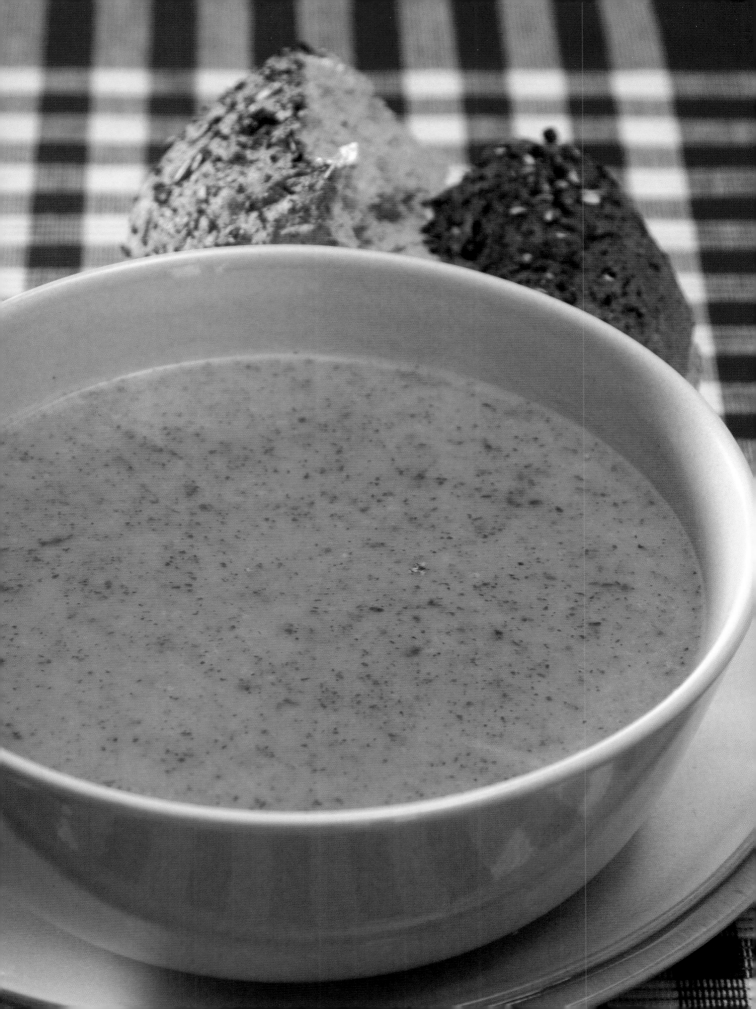

# Watercress & Potato Soup

*One Pot*

A delicious nutritious soup that takes only minutes to make.

## Serves 2

**1 tbsp olive oil**
**1 onion, peeled and chopped**
**225g/8oz potatoes, peeled
    and chopped**
**50g/2oz bunch watercress**
**300ml/½pt stock**
**150ml/¼pt semi-skimmed
    milk**
**small pinch freshly grated
    nutmeg**

## Serves 4

**2 tbsp olive oil**
**2 onions, peeled and
    chopped**
**450g/1lb potatoes, peeled
    and chopped**
**100g/4oz bunch watercress**
**600ml/1pt stock**
**300ml/½pt semi-skimmed
    milk**
**pinch freshly grated nutmeg**

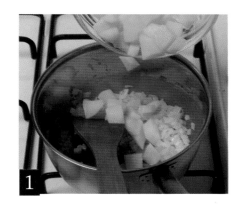

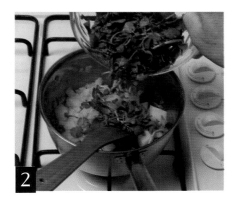

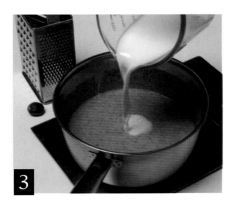

1 Heat the oil in a large saucepan and cook the onion over a moderate heat until it becomes softened. Add the potatoes and cook, covered, for 5 minutes, shaking the pan from time to time.

2 Wash the watercress and chop roughly. Add to the pan, stirring to mix. Add the stock and bring gently to the boil.

3 Reduce the heat to a gentle simmer, cover the pan and cook for 15 minutes, until the potatoes are tender. Remove the pan from the heat and allow the soup to cool for 10 minutes. Blend in a food processor or blender until smooth and then return to the pan. Stir in the milk and nutmeg, and gently reheat until piping hot. Serve.

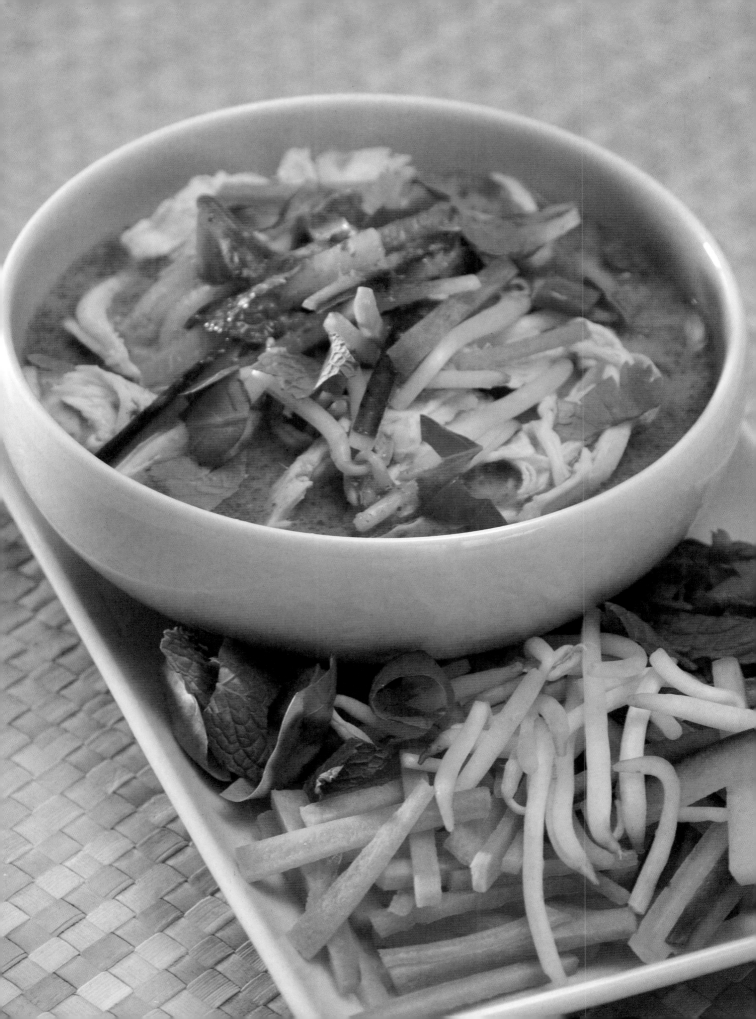

# Chicken Laksa

*Family Favourite*

Don't be put off by the list of ingredients. This delicious soup is a meal in a bowl that you build at the table to your own tastes.

*Serves 2*

½ stick lemon grass
½ red chilli
½ clove garlic
1cm/½in piece fresh ginger
1 shallot
¼ tsp turmeric
4 tbsp coriander leaves
¼ tsp tamarind paste
1 tbsp peanut oil
50g/2oz noodles
1 large chicken breast,
   cooked
50g/2oz cucumber
50g/2oz carrot
40g/1½oz bean sprouts
½ tbsp fresh basil
½ tbsp fresh mint
225ml/8fl oz chicken stock
100ml/3½fl oz coconut milk
½ tbsp nam pla (fish sauce)

*Serves 4*

1 stick lemon grass
1 red chilli
1 clove garlic
2.5cm/1in piece fresh ginger
2 shallots
½ tsp turmeric
8 tbsp coriander leaves
½ tsp tamarind paste
2 tbsp peanut oil
100g/4oz noodles
2 large chicken breasts,
   cooked
100g/4oz cucumber
100g/4oz carrot
75g/3oz bean sprouts
1 tbsp fresh basil
1 tbsp fresh mint
450ml/¾pt chicken stock
200ml/7fl oz coconut milk
1 tbsp nam pla (fish sauce)

1 First make up the spice paste. Remove the tough outer layers from the lemon grass and discard, then chop the tender middle part and place in a food processor. Roughly chop the red chilli, removing the seeds if you prefer less heat. Peel the garlic, ginger and shallots and roughly chop. Add these to the food processor along with the turmeric, 2 (4) tbsp of the coriander leaves, the tamarind paste, ½ (1) tbsp of the oil and 1 (2) tbsp water. Process until the mixture forms a rough paste. Scoop into a bowl and set to one side.

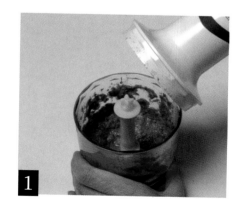

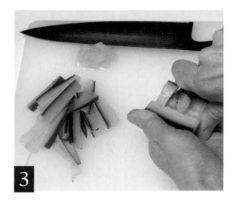

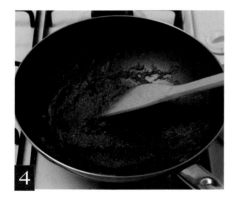

2 Cook the noodles according to the pack instructions, then drain and set to one side. Shred the chicken breast and set to one side.

3 Deseed the cucumber and then cut the flesh into matchsticks. Peel the carrot and cut into matchsticks. Arrange these on a serving plate along with the bean sprouts. Roughly chop the basil, mint and remaining coriander and add to the plate.

4 Heat the remaining oil in a large saucepan or wok and cook the spice paste over a moderate heat until it starts to change colour. Now add the chicken stock, coconut milk and nam pla. Bring gently to the boil.

5 Divide the noodles between the serving bowls, and then top with the prepared chicken. Once the stock mixture is boiling, pour it over the noodles and chicken. Serve with the plate of vegetables and herbs to be added as desired.

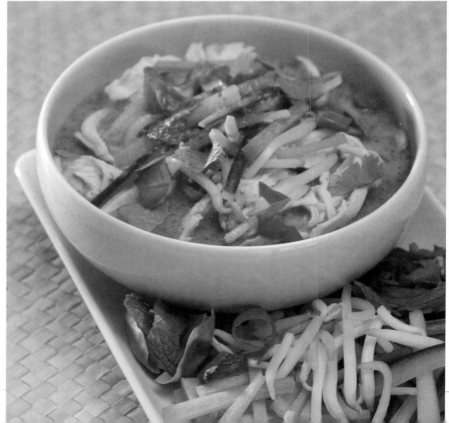

# Squid with Avocado Salsa

## Easy Entertaining

Squid is low in saturated fat and high in protein. It is also a good source of vitamin B6 and B12. Avocados give us potassium, which helps to control blood pressure.

### Serves 2

1 small ripe avocado
½ lime
2 tomatoes
½ green chilli
3 tbsp fresh coriander, chopped
150g/5oz small squid, cleaned
1 tsp sunflower oil
salad leaves to serve

### Serves 4

1 large ripe avocado
1 lime
4 tomatoes
1 green chilli
6 tbsp fresh coriander, chopped
300g/10½oz small squid, cleaned
2 tsp sunflower oil
salad leaves to serve

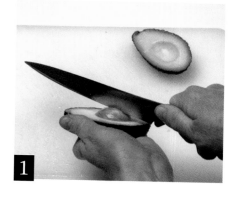

1

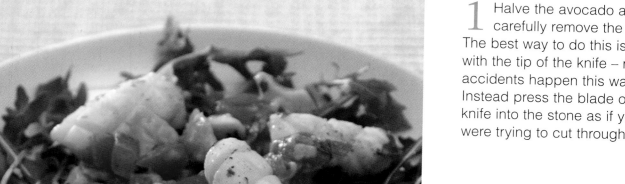

1 Halve the avocado and carefully remove the stone. The best way to do this is not with the tip of the knife – many accidents happen this way. Instead press the blade of the knife into the stone as if you were trying to cut through it.

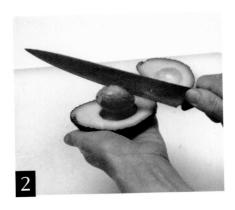

2

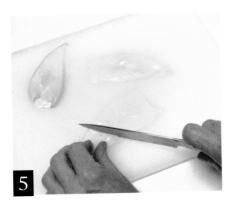

5

2 Give the knife a slight twist and the stone should just lift straight out on the blade of the knife.

3 Remove the peel and chop the flesh into small dice. Place in a glass or plastic mixing bowl. Squeeze the juice from the lime and add to the avocado, tossing well to mix.

4 Deseed the tomatoes and chop, then add to the avocado. Finely chop the chilli, deseeding it if you do not like things too spicy. Add the coriander and mix well, then set to one side while you cook the squid.

5 Wash and dry the squid, then cut in half and score the skin diagonally. Place in a bowl, drizzle over the oil and toss to coat.

6 Heat a griddle pan over a high heat and cook the squid for 3–4 minutes, turning halfway through.

7 To serve, divide the squid between 2 (4) plates, accompanied by a large spoonful of the salsa and a few salad leaves.

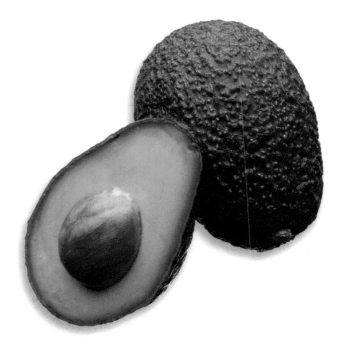

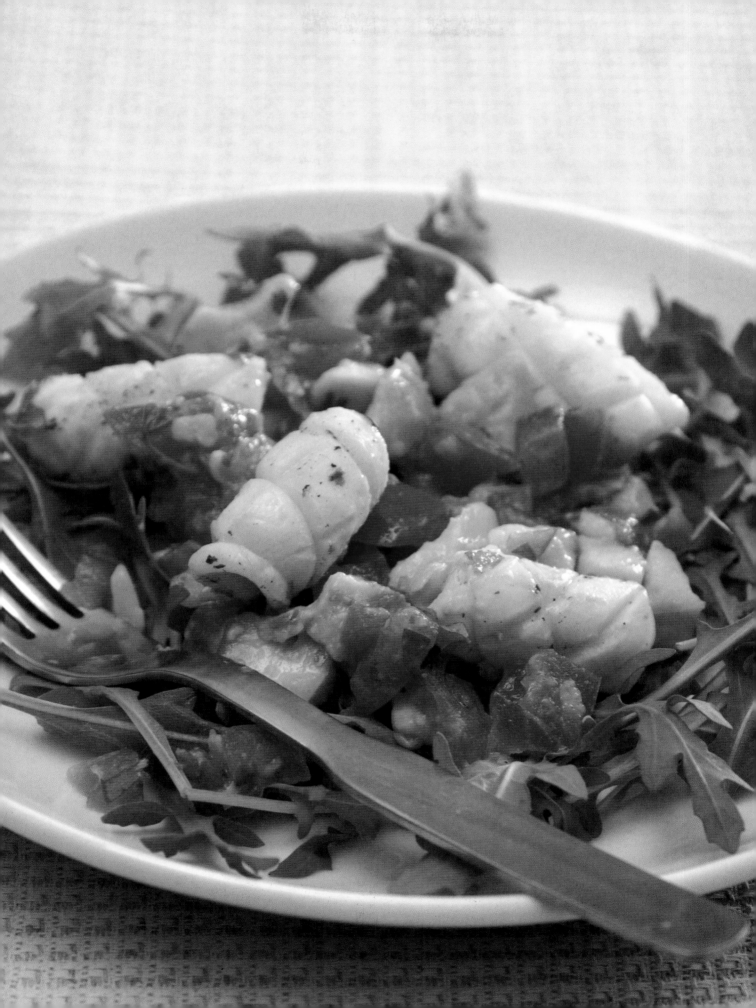

# Mushroom & Pepper Pâté

## Easy Entertaining

Pâté is usually quite calorific owing to its fat content. This is a light and tasty version that is also suitable for vegetarians.

### Serves 2

½ red pepper
15g/½oz unsalted butter
1 small clove garlic, peeled and crushed
200g/7oz button mushrooms, finely chopped
2 tbsp cream cheese
1 tbsp fresh parsley, chopped
salt and freshly ground black pepper
toast to serve

### Serves 4

1 red pepper
25g/1oz unsalted butter
1 clove garlic, peeled and crushed
400g/14oz button mushrooms, finely chopped
4 tbsp cream cheese
2 tbsp fresh parsley, chopped
salt and freshly ground black pepper
toast to serve

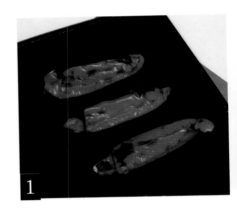

1

1 Preheat the grill to high. Deseed the pepper and cut into thick strips. Place under the preheated grill and cook until the skin becomes blackened and charred. Remove, place in a small bowl and cover with cling film. Set to one side for 15 minutes. Then peel and finely chop.

2 Melt the butter in a large saucepan and cook the garlic over a gentle heat for 1–2 minutes.

3 Add the mushrooms and chopped pepper, stirring well to mix. Cook for 5 minutes until the mushrooms start to soften.

4 Reduce the heat to a gentle simmer and cook uncovered, stirring from time to time, until the mixture is looking dry. Remove from the heat and leave to cool fully.

5 Beat in the cream cheese. Stir through the parsley. Season to taste before serving with fresh toast.

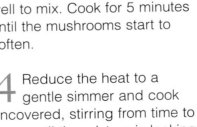

3

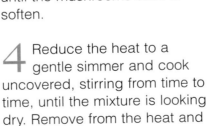

5

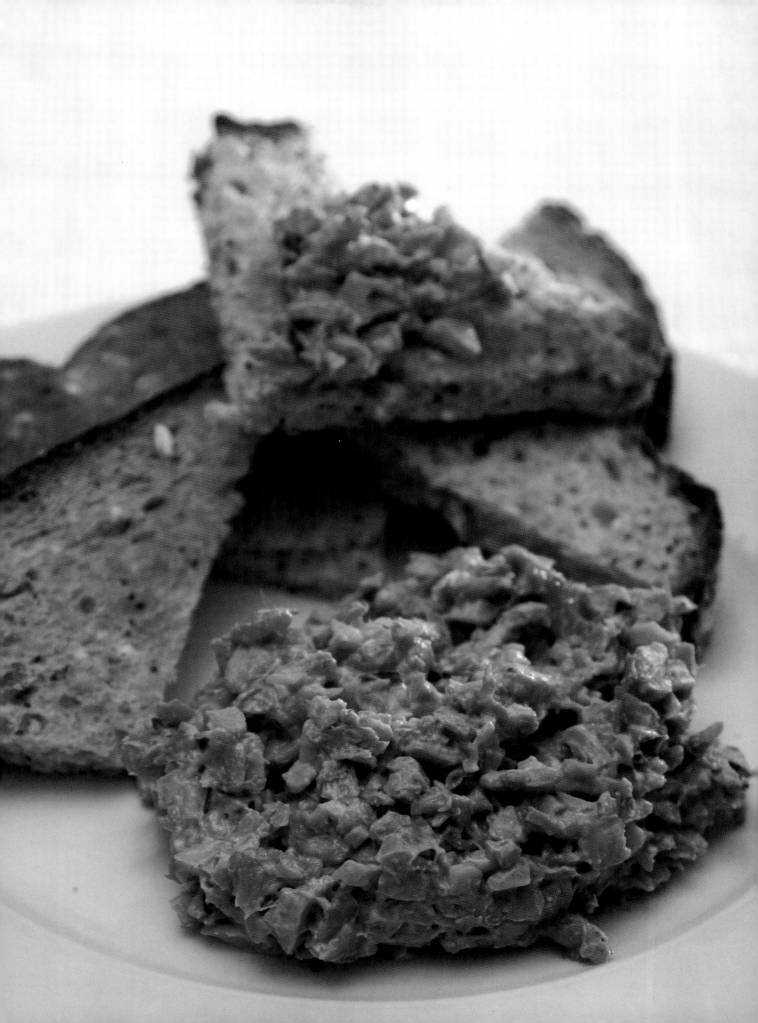

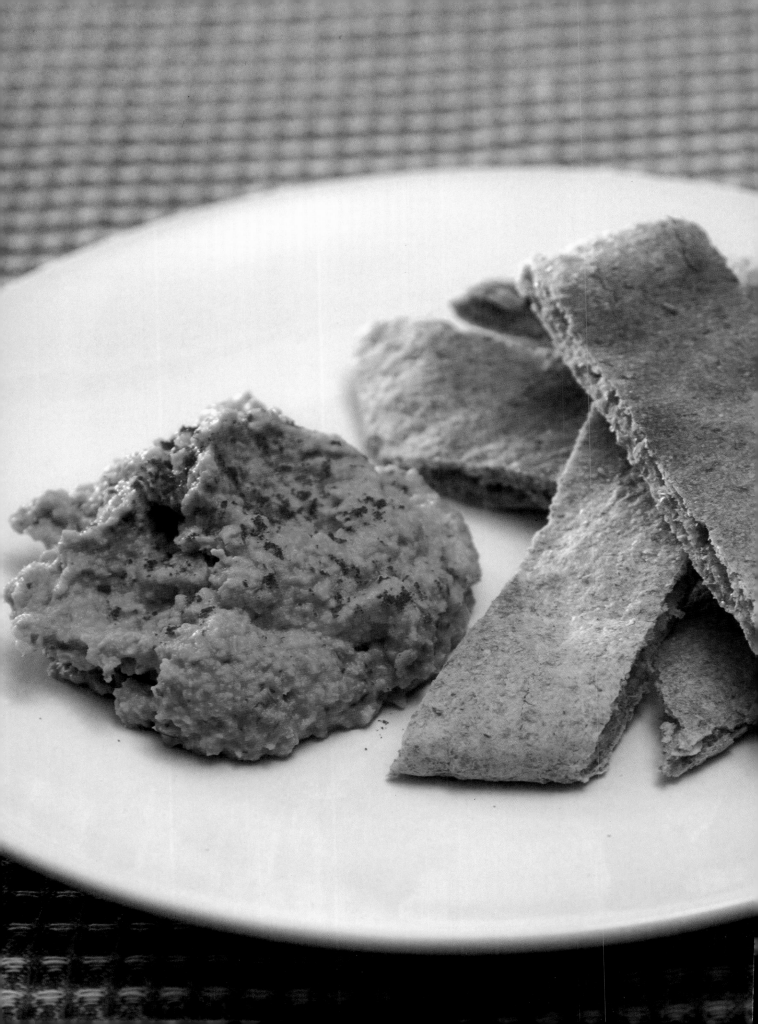

# Green Dip

*Quick and Easy*

This dip uses unusual ingredients and it really is delicious.

## Serves 2

90g/3½oz frozen petit pois
2 tsp olive oil
1 small clove garlic, finely
   chopped
½ small onion, finely
   chopped
1cm/½in fresh ginger,
   peeled and finely grated
4 tbsp coriander, chopped
2 tbsp plain yoghurt
salt and freshly ground
   pepper
small pinch of cayenne
   pepper
pitta bread or crudités to
   serve

## Serves 4

175g/6oz frozen petit pois
4 tsp olive oil
1 clove garlic, finely chopped
1 small onion, finely
   chopped
2.5cm/1in fresh ginger,
   peeled and finely grated
8 tbsp coriander, chopped
4 tbsp plain yoghurt
salt and freshly ground
   pepper
pinch of cayenne pepper
pitta bread or crudités to
   serve

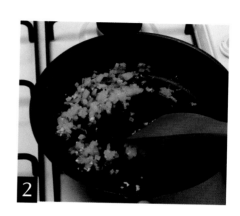

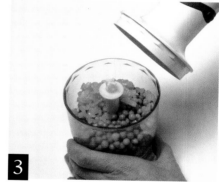

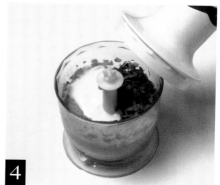

1 Cook the petit pois according to the packet instructions, then drain and set to one side.

2 Heat the oil in a small frying pan and cook the onion and garlic over a moderate heat until they are softened but not golden. Add the ginger and cook for 1–2 minutes more, stirring well to mix. Remove from the heat.

3 Place the peas and onion mixture in a food processor or blender and process until almost smooth.

4 Add the coriander and yoghurt and process briefly to mix.

5 Turn out into a serving dish. Season lightly with salt and freshly ground pepper, and sprinkle with a pinch of cayenne pepper. Serve with toasted pitta bread or crudités.

# Spiced Parsnip Sticks with Yoghurt Dip

*children's choice*

Parsnips cut into sticks and roasted are sweet and tasty – there never quite seems to be enough!

## Serves 2

**250g/9oz parsnips, peeled**
**1 tbsp oil**
**2 tsp smoked paprika**
**100ml/3½fl oz plain yoghurt**
**1 small clove garlic, peeled and crushed**
**2 tbsp fresh mint, chopped**
**1 tsp olive oil**
**salt and freshly ground black pepper**

## Serves 4

**500g/1lb 2oz parsnips, peeled**
**2 tbsp oil**
**4 tsp smoked paprika**
**200ml/7fl oz plain yoghurt**
**1 clove garlic, peeled and crushed**
**4 tbsp fresh mint, chopped**
**2 tsp olive oil**
**salt and freshly ground black pepper**

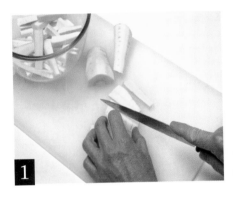

1 Preheat the oven to 220°C/425°F/Gas Mark 7. Using a sharp knife, cut the parsnips into thin sticks. Place the sticks in a mixing bowl, drizzle over the oil and toss to coat thoroughly.

2 Sprinkle with the paprika and mix again. Line a large baking tray with non-stick parchment paper.

3 Spread the spiced parsnip sticks in a single layer over the lined baking tray. Cook for about 35 minutes, turning once halfway, until golden and cooked through.

4 While the parsnips are cooking, pour the yoghurt into a mixing bowl and add the garlic, mint and olive oil. Stir well to combine, season to taste and serve with the spiced wedges.

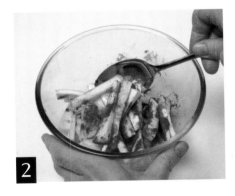

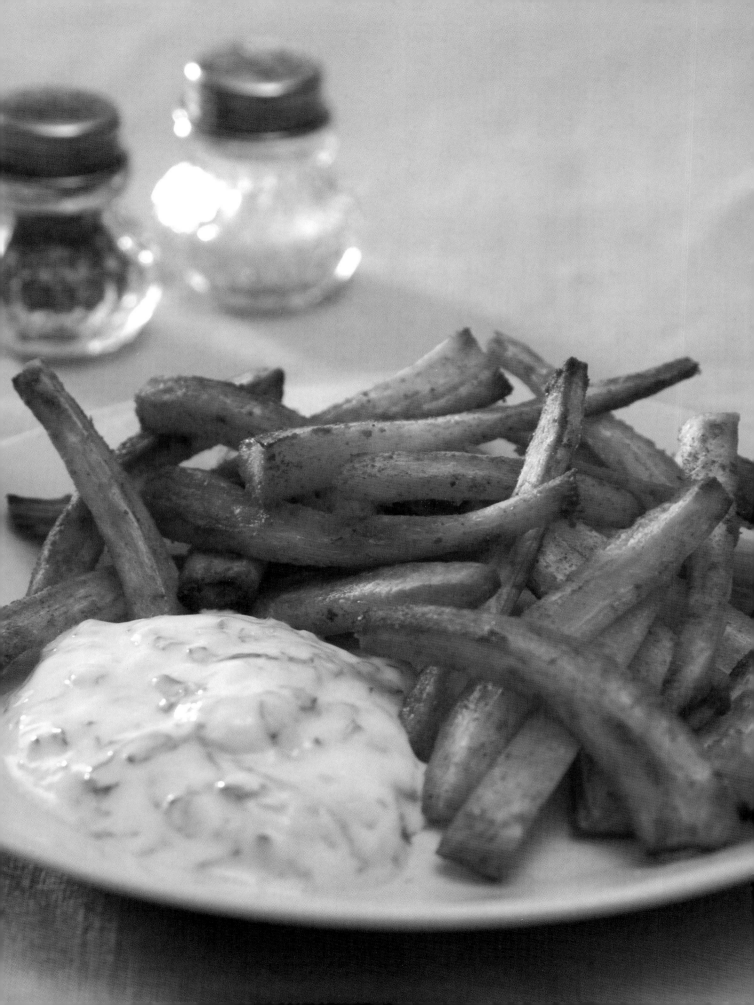

# Mackerel Pâté

*Easy Entertaining*

Mackerel is a good source of omega-3 fatty acids, as it is classed as an oily fish.

## Serves 2

100g/4oz ricotta
1 tbsp creamed horseradish
100g/4oz smoked mackerel
  fillets
¼ tsp freshly ground black
  pepper
1 tbsp parsley, chopped
brown bread toasted to serve

## Serves 4

225g/8oz ricotta
2 tbsp creamed horseradish
225g/8oz smoked mackerel
  fillets
½ tsp freshly ground black
  pepper
2 tbsp parsley, chopped
brown bread toasted to serve

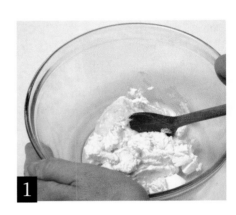

1 Place the ricotta and horseradish in a mixing bowl and, using a wooden spoon, beat well until mixed and smooth.

2 Remove the skin from the fish and, using your fingers, flake it into the mixing bowl. At this point it is a good idea to make sure all the bones have been removed from the fillets.

3 Stir well to mix. Add the black pepper and parsley and stir again. Serve with toasted brown bread and a small salad. This is also good as a sandwich filling and will keep in the fridge for two days.

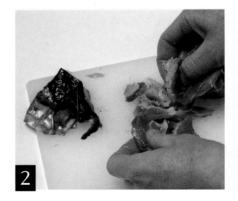

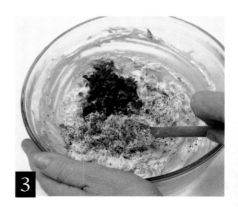

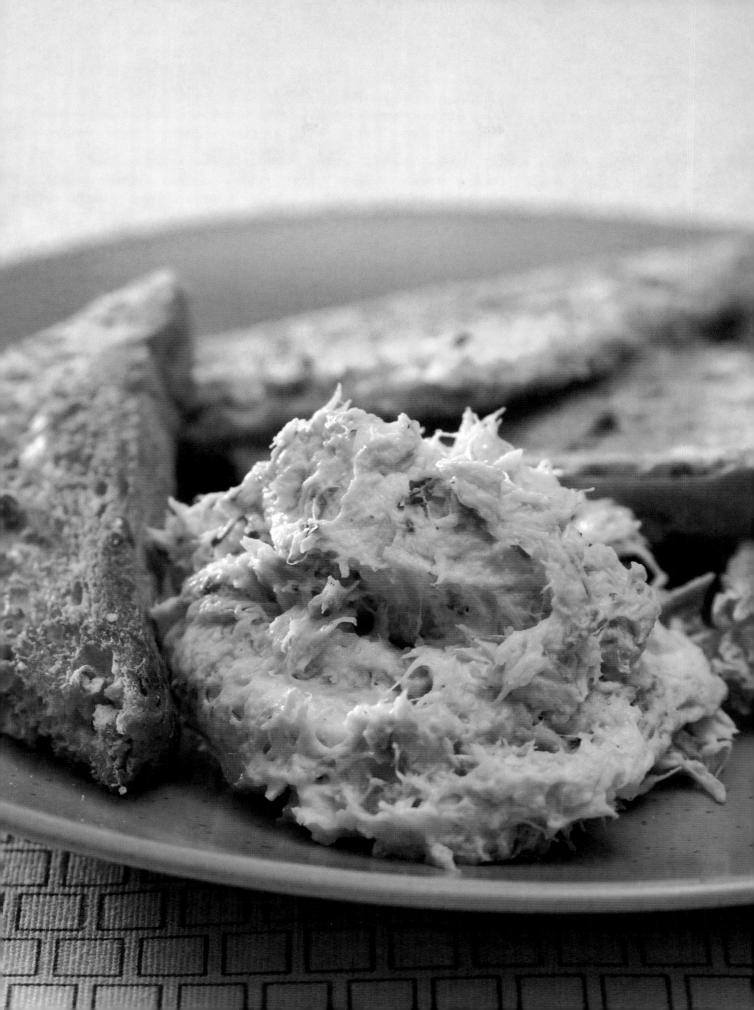

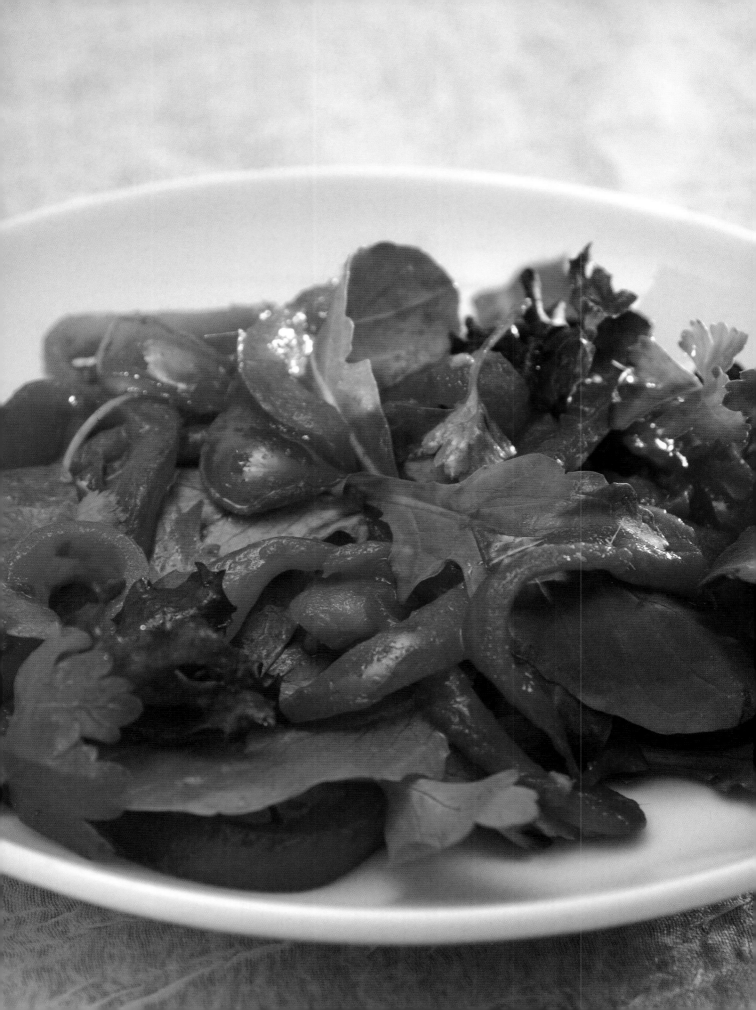

# Pepper & Anchovy Salad

*Easy Entertaining*

Peppers are high in vitamin C.

## Serves 2

**2 red peppers**
**1 tsp olive oil**
**4 anchovies in oil**
**1 small clove garlic**
**50g/2oz salad leaves**

## Serves 4

**4 red peppers**
**2 tsp olive oil**
**8 anchovies in oil**
**1 clove garlic**
**100g/ 4oz salad leaves**

1 Using a vegetable peeler, peel the red peppers. You won't be able to remove all the skin – just remove as much as possible.

2 Halve and deseed the peppers, then cut them into long, thin strips.

3 Heat the oil in a frying pan over a moderate heat and cook the pepper strips for 20 minutes, stirring from time to time, until tender.

4 Using kitchen paper, blot the anchovies of any excess oil. Add them to the pan along with the garlic and 2 (4) tbsp water. Cook, stirring.

5 When the water has evaporated and the anchovies have melted into a smooth paste, remove from the heat.

6 Place the salad leaves in a bowl and add the contents of the frying pan. Toss to mix and divide between the serving plates. Serve immediately.

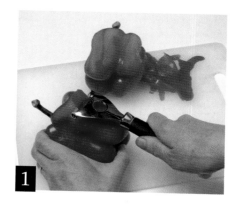

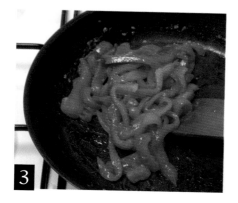

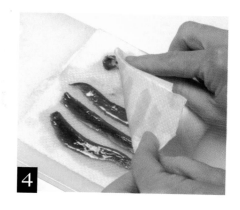

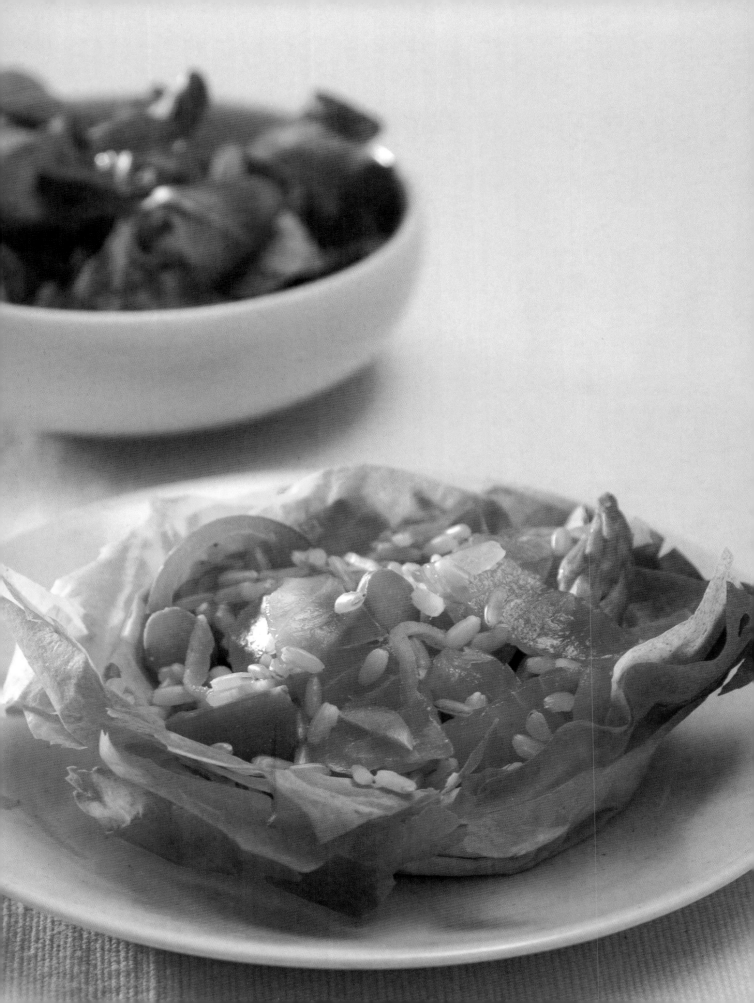

# Smoked Salmon & Wasabi Tarts

*Easy Entertaining*

Light crisp tarts filled with spiced rice, asparagus, tomatoes and smoked salmon.

### Serves 2

**2 sheets filo pastry**
**olive oil for spraying**
**50g/2oz brown rice**
**¼ tsp wasabi paste**
**½ tbsp pickled ginger, sliced**
**2 asparagus tips**
**4 cherry tomatoes**
**50g/2oz smoked salmon**

### Serves 4

**4 sheets filo pastry**
**olive oil for spraying**
**100g/4oz brown rice**
**½ tsp wasabi paste**
**1 tbsp pickled ginger, sliced**
**4 asparagus tips**
**8 cherry tomatoes**
**100g/4oz smoked salmon**

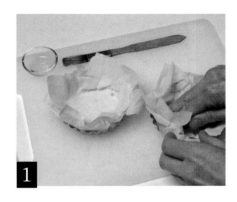

1 Preheat the oven to 200°C/400°F/Gas Mark 6. Cut the filo pastry into 8 (16), 15cm/6in squares. Spray each piece lightly with oil and then divide between 2 (4) individual 10cm/4in tartlet tins, pressing gently into place and leaving the edges hanging over the tin. Bake in the preheated oven for 15 minutes until golden. Remove and set to one side.

2 Cook the rice according to the packet instructions, then drain and stir through the wasabi and ginger.

3 Bring a pan of water to the boil and cook the asparagus for 4 minutes, then drain. When cool enough to handle, chop the asparagus into bite-size pieces. Cut the tomatoes into quarters and slice the salmon into thin strips.

4 Toss the salmon, asparagus and tomatoes through the rice. Divide the mixture between the tartlet cases and serve.

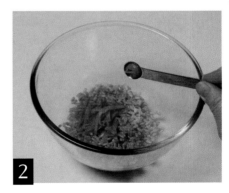

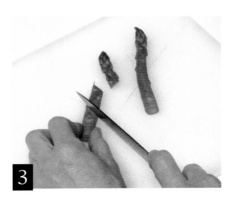

# Grilled Tomato Salad

*Quick and Easy*

Studies have shown tomatoes to be excellent in helping to protect from some forms of cancer.

### Serves 2

25g/1oz fresh brown
  breadcrumbs
1 tbsp Parmesan cheese,
  finely grated
1 small clove garlic, peeled
  and crushed
2 tbsp fresh parsley
¼ tsp lemon zest
4 ripe tomatoes, halved
salad leaves to serve
2 tsp balsamic vinegar

### Serves 4

50g/2oz fresh brown
  breadcrumbs
2 tbsp Parmesan cheese,
  finely grated
1 clove garlic, peeled and
  crushed
4 tbsp fresh parsley
½ tsp lemon zest
8 ripe tomatoes, halved
salad leaves to serve
4 tsp balsamic vinegar

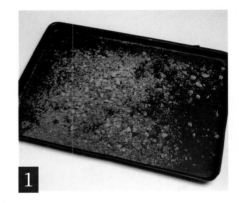

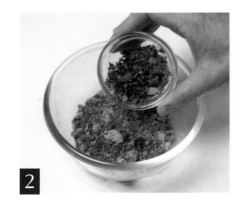

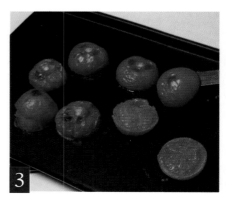

1 Preheat the oven to 200°C/400°F/Gas Mark 6. In a mixing bowl stir the breadcrumbs, Parmesan cheese and garlic together. Spread the mixture in a thin layer over a non-stick baking tray and cook in the preheated oven for 10 minutes until golden and crisp.

2 Preheat the grill to high. Tip the toasted breadcrumbs back into the mixing bowl. Chop the parsley and add to the breadcrumb mixture with the lemon zest and stir well to mix.

3 Cook the tomatoes under the preheated grill, turning once, until tender and cooked through. Arrange the salad leaves on serving plates and top with the cooked tomatoes. Sprinkle with the balsamic vinegar and then top with the breadcrumb mixture to serve.

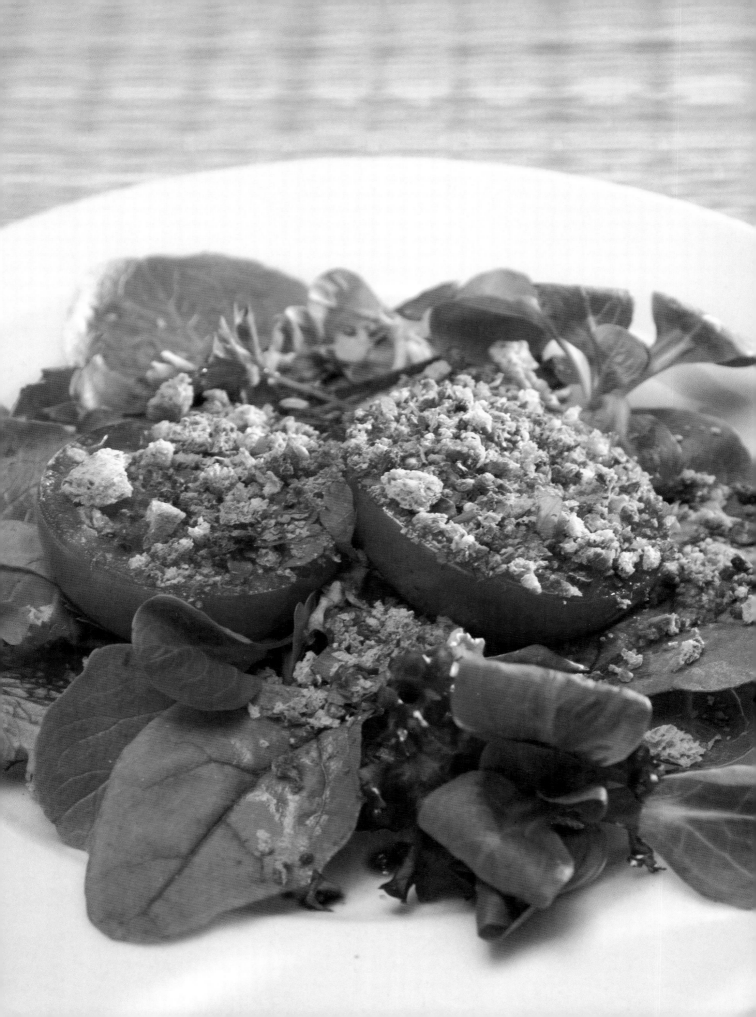

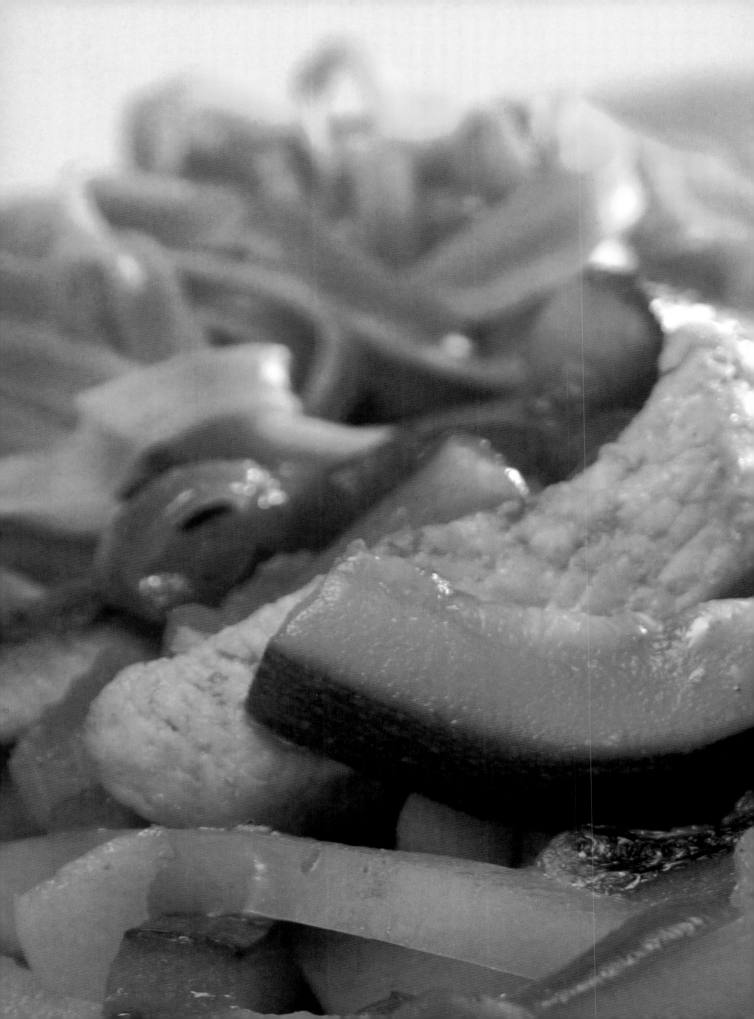

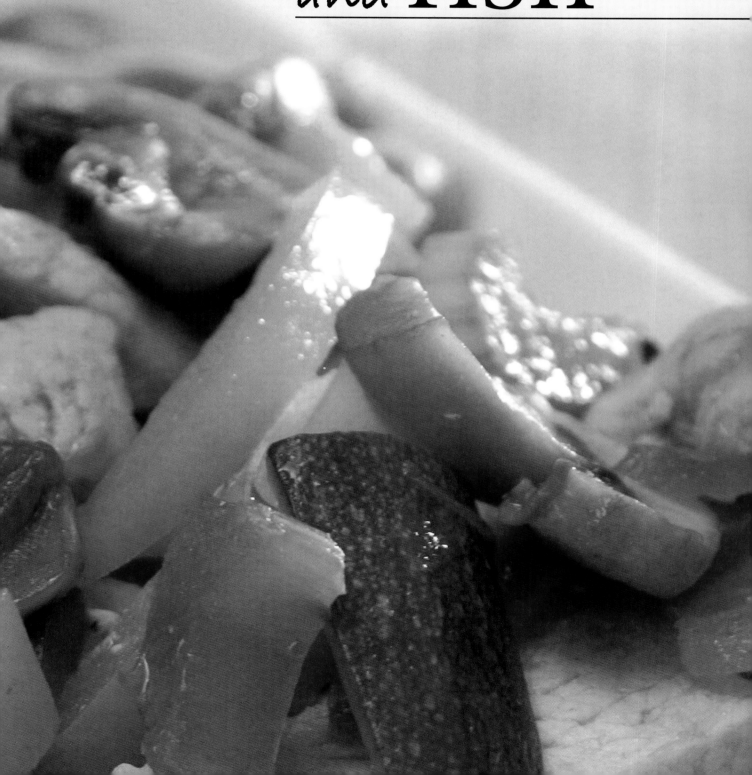

# meat and fish

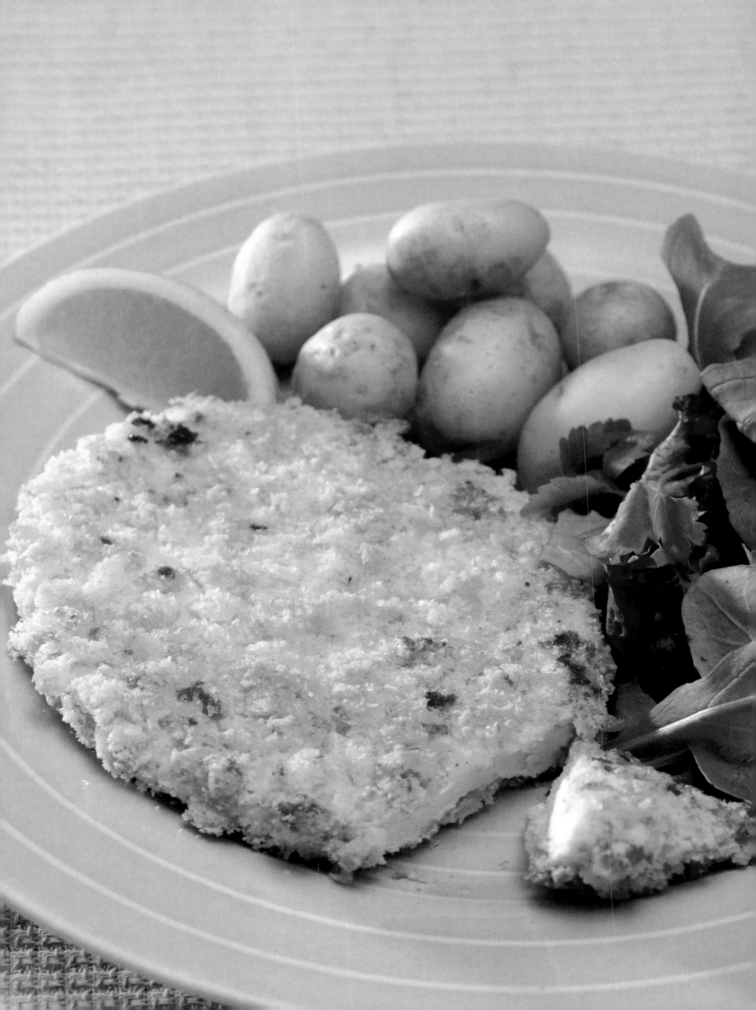

# Chicken Escalope

*Family Favourite*

Traditionally these are fried, however they are just as good baked in the oven until golden and crisp. Chicken is an excellent form of protein and vitamin A and is also low in fat.

### Serves 2

**2 skinless, boneless chicken breasts**
**50g/2oz stale white bread**
**2 tbsp Parmesan cheese, freshly grated**
**1 egg**
**2 tbsp wholemeal flour**
**new potatoes, salad and lemon wedges to serve**

### Serves 4

**4 skinless, boneless chicken breasts**
**100g/4oz stale white bread**
**4 tbsp Parmesan cheese, freshly grated**
**2 eggs**
**4 tbsp wholemeal flour**
**new potatoes, salad and lemon wedges to serve**

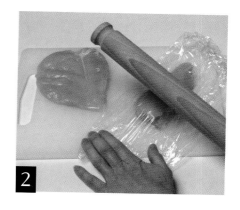

1 Preheat the oven to 200°C/400°F/Gas Mark 6. Line a shallow baking tray with parchment paper and set to one side.

2 Take one chicken breast at a time and place between two sheets of cling film. Using a rolling pin, beat the chicken breast until it is approximately 1cm/½in thick. Repeat with the remaining chicken breasts.

3 Remove the crusts from the bread and discard. Roughly chop the bread, place in a food processor or blender and process until the bread becomes coarse crumbs. Mix in the Parmesan cheese and then tip onto a large plate.

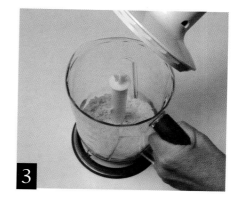

4 Beat the egg and pour into a shallow bowl. Taking one chicken breast at a time, dust it first with the flour, shaking off any excess, then dip it in the egg. Now press it into the breadcrumb mixture to coat it evenly. Place on the prepared baking tray and repeat with the remaining pieces of chicken.

5 Cook in the preheated oven for about 15 minutes, until golden, crisp and cooked through. Serve with boiled new potatoes, salad and lemon wedges for squeezing.

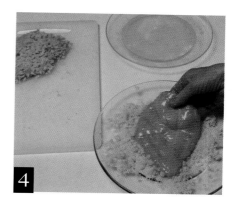

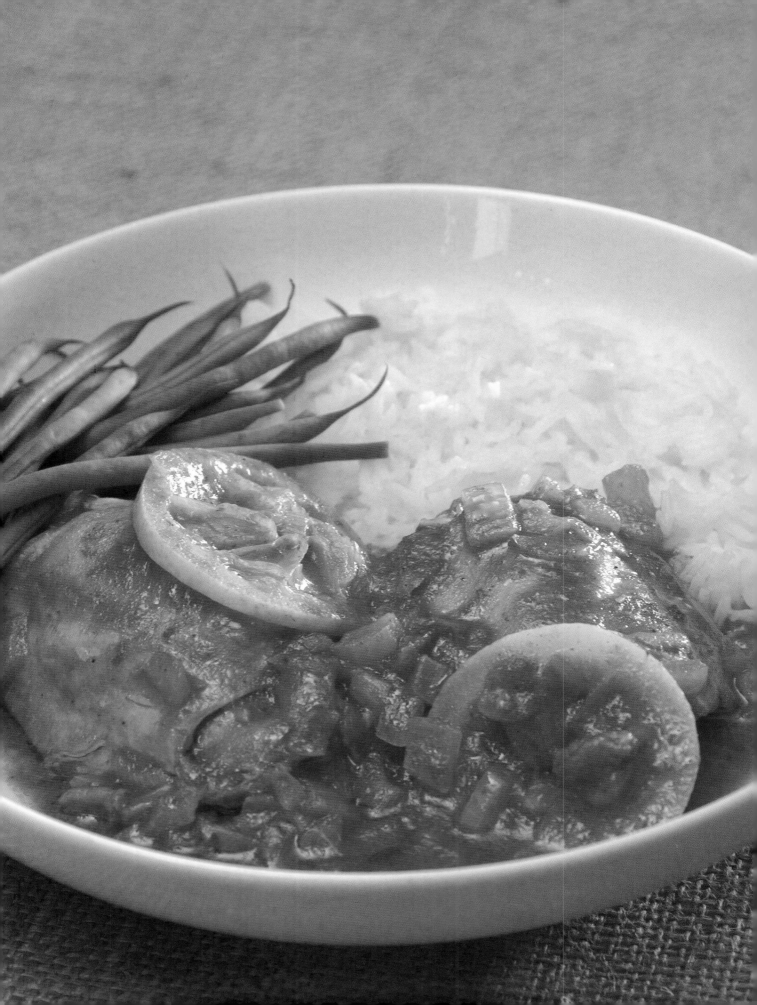

# Lemon Chicken Curry

*One Pot*

By removing the skin from the chicken, you remove almost all of the fat.

## Serves 2

**4 small chicken portions**
**1 tbsp sunflower oil**
**1 onion, peeled and chopped**
**1 clove garlic, peeled and crushed**
**1 tbsp curry powder**
**2 tbsp tomato purée**
**½ lemon, sliced**
**1 tbsp flour**
**300ml/½pt chicken stock**
**rice and vegetables to serve**

## Serves 4

**8 small chicken portions**
**2 tbsp sunflower oil**
**1 large onion, peeled and chopped**
**2 cloves garlic, peeled and crushed**
**2 tbsp curry powder**
**4 tbsp tomato purée**
**1 lemon, sliced**
**2 tbsp flour**
**600ml/1pt chicken stock**
**rice and vegetables to serve**

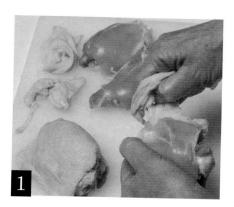

1 Remove the skin from the chicken pieces and discard. Heat the oil in a frying pan and cook the onion and garlic over a moderate heat until softened.

2 Add the chicken pieces and cook for about 6 minutes, turning to brown all over. Stir in the curry powder and cook for 1 minute.

3 Add the tomato purée and the lemon slices to the pan and stir to mix. Place the flour in a small bowl and add enough of the chicken stock to form a smooth paste. Stir in the remaining stock and add to the pan, mixing thoroughly.

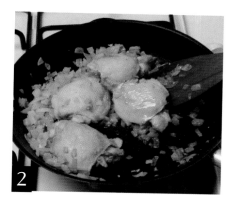

4 Bring to the boil, then reduce the heat to a gentle simmer. Cover the pan with a well-fitting lid and cook undisturbed for 25 minutes. Serve with rice and a vegetable of your choice.

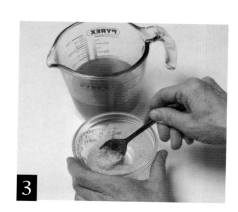

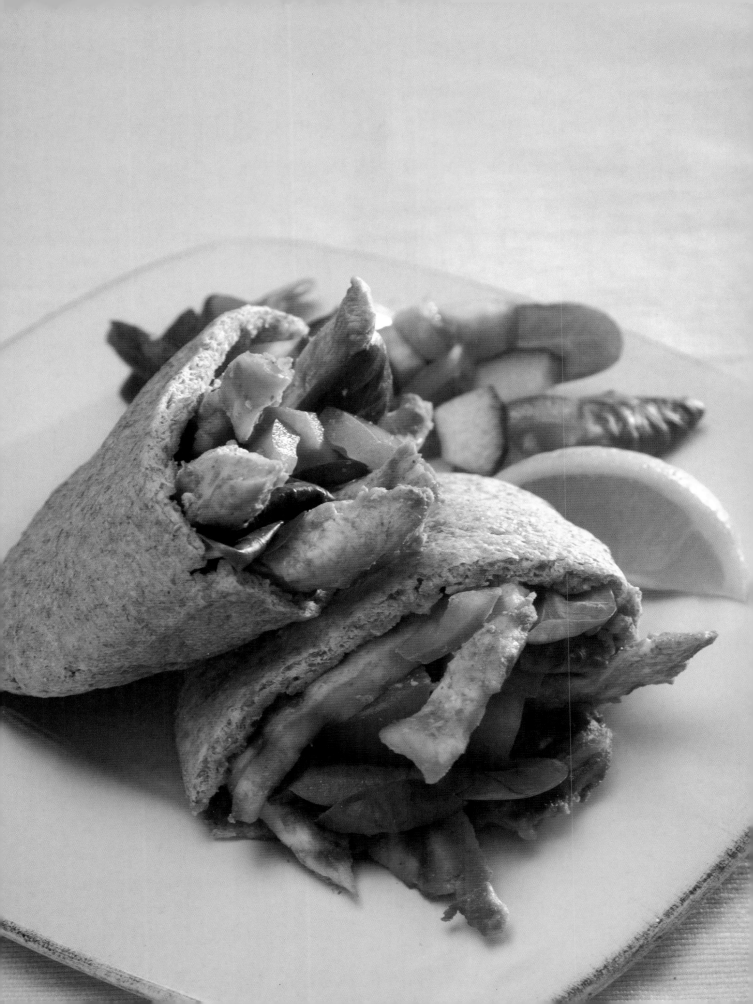

# Moroccan Chicken in Pittas

*Family Favourite*

Spiced chicken and salad in pitta breads are as popular in winter as they are in summer.

### Serves 2

2 skinless, boneless chicken breasts
1 lemon
½ tbsp olive oil
1 tsp ground cumin
½ tsp ground turmeric
¼ tsp chilli powder
1 clove garlic, peeled and crushed
¼ cucumber
2 tomatoes
1 tbsp fresh mint leaves
1 tbsp fresh coriander leaves
2 wholemeal pitta breads
50g/2oz salad leaves

### Serves 4

4 skinless, boneless chicken breasts
2 lemons
1 tbsp olive oil
2 tsp ground cumin
1 tsp ground turmeric
½ tsp chilli powder
2 cloves garlic, peeled and crushed
½ cucumber
4 tomatoes
2 tbsp fresh mint leaves
2 tbsp fresh coriander leaves
4 wholemeal pitta breads
100g/4oz salad leaves

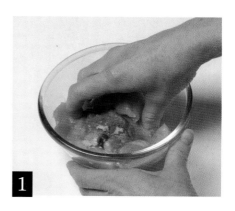

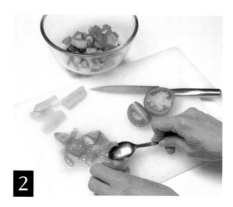

1 Slice the chicken breasts into thin strips and place in a glass or plastic bowl. Squeeze the juice from half the lemon and add to the chicken along with the oil, cumin, turmeric, chilli powder and garlic. Use your hands to knead the chicken well to mix. Cover with cling film and leave in the fridge to marinate for at least 2 hours or up to 12 hours if possible.

2 Make up the salad. Halve the cucumber lengthways and, using a teaspoon, remove the seeds and discard. Dice the cucumber and place in a plastic or glass bowl. Halve and deseed the tomatoes, cut into dice and add to the cucumber. Roughly tear the mint and coriander leaves and add to the cucumber and tomato, toss to mix.

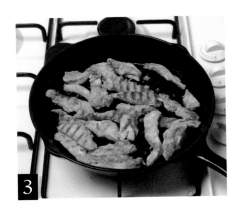

3 When you are ready to start cooking, preheat a griddle pan over a moderate heat. Remove the chicken from the marinade and cook in the preheated pan for 6–8 minutes, turning once, until golden brown and cooked through.

4 Warm the pitta breads under the grill. Split them open and stuff with the salad leaves. Top with some of the cucumber and tomato salad, followed by the chicken strips. Cut the remaining lemon into wedges and squeeze a little juice over each chicken-stuffed pitta. Serve accompanied by the remaining salad.

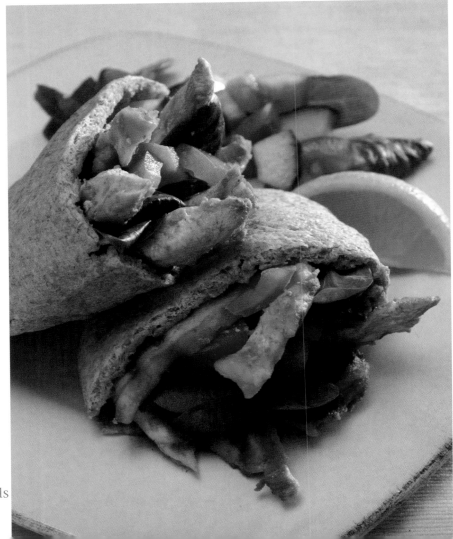

# Wrapped Chicken with Orange & Almonds

*Easy Entertaining*

Wrapping the chicken and vegetables in baking parchment parcels and baking them in the oven is a perfect low-fat way to cook.

## Serves 2

- 100g/4oz green beans, trimmed
- 100g/4oz carrots, peeled and cut into batons
- 2 chicken breasts
- ½ large orange
- 1 garlic clove, peeled and crushed
- 1 tbsp fresh parsley, chopped
- 2 tsp olive oil
- 2 shallots, peeled and finely chopped
- ½ tbsp cornflour
- 2 tbsp almonds, flaked and toasted

## Serves 4

- 200g/7oz green beans, trimmed
- 200g/7oz carrots, peeled and cut into batons
- 4 chicken breasts
- 1 large orange
- 2 garlic cloves, peeled and crushed
- 2 tbsp fresh parsley, chopped
- 4 tsp olive oil
- 4 shallots, peeled and finely chopped
- 1 tbsp cornflour
- 4 tbsp almonds, flaked and toasted

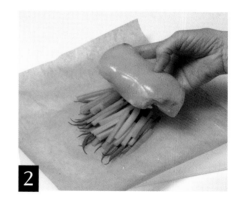

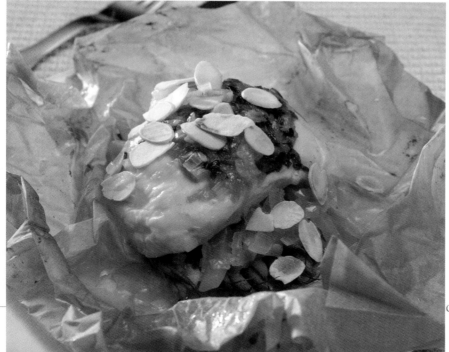

1 Preheat the oven to 200°C/400°F/Gas Mark 6. Take 2 (4) large squares of baking parchment and divide the beans equally between each piece, arranging them in the centre.

2 Top the beans with the carrot batons, followed by a chicken breast.

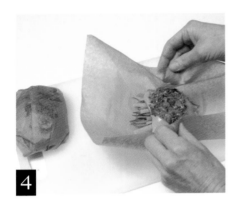

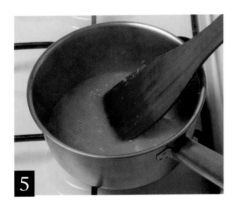

3 Remove the zest from the orange and place in a mixing bowl. Add the garlic, parsley and half the oil. Mix thoroughly then divide this mixture between each chicken breast and spread thinly to cover the breast.

4 Pull the parchment paper up over the chicken and vegetables and fold the edges together to seal securely. Place on a baking tray and cook in the preheated oven for 25 minutes.

5 Heat the remaining oil in a small saucepan and add the chopped shallots. Cook over a gentle heat until they become softened. Squeeze the juice from the orange and add to the saucepan.

6 Blend the cornflour with ½ (1) tbsp cold water until it forms a smooth paste. Add to the saucepan, stirring well to mix. Bring gently to the boil and cook, stirring, until the mixture thickens.

7 Remove the chicken from the oven. Place each parcel on a serving plate and open the paper. Scatter over the toasted almonds and serve, accompanied by the orange sauce.

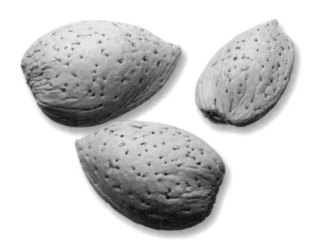

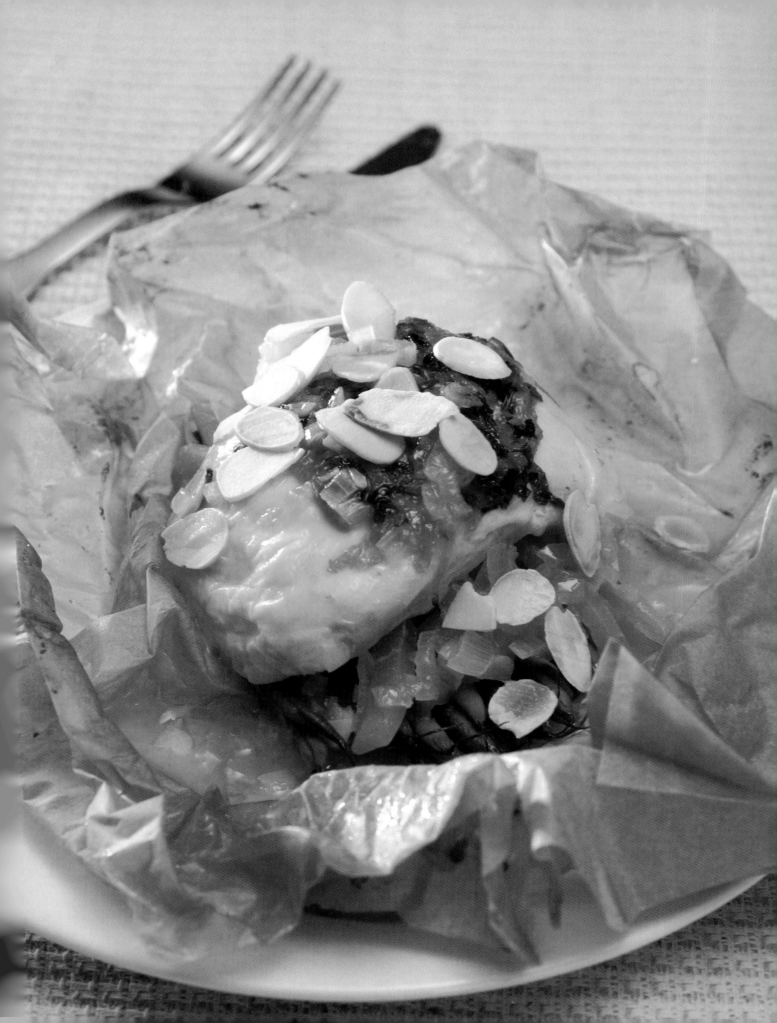

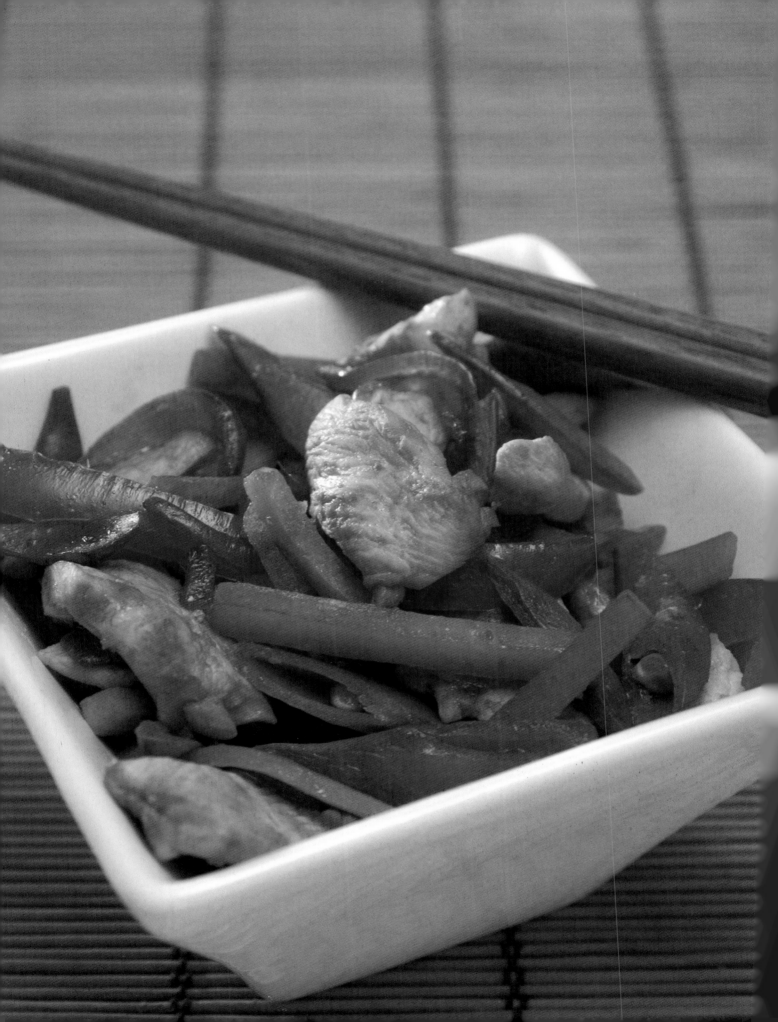

# Ginger & Lemon Chicken

## *Family Favourite*

Chicken breast is a wonderful form of protein, and simply by removing the skin you remove most of the fat.

### Serves 2

**2 tsp olive oil**
**1 small red onion, peeled**
   **and thinly sliced**
**½ red pepper, deseeded**
   **and cut into strips**
**1 carrot, peeled and cut into**
   **matchsticks**
**2 skinless chicken breasts**
**75g/3oz sugar snaps,**
   **trimmed and sliced**
**1 piece stem ginger, thinly**
   **sliced**
**1 tbsp stem ginger syrup**
**½ lemon**
**1 tbsp soy sauce**
**brown rice to serve**

### Serves 4

**4 tsp olive oil**
**1 red onion, peeled and thinly**
   **sliced**
**1 red pepper, deseeded and**
   **cut into strips**
**2 carrots, peeled and cut into**
   **matchsticks**
**4 skinless chicken breasts**
**150g/5oz sugar snaps,**
   **trimmed and sliced**
**2 pieces stem ginger, thinly**
   **sliced**
**2 tbsp stem ginger syrup**
**1 lemon**
**2 tbsp soy sauce**
**brown rice to serve**

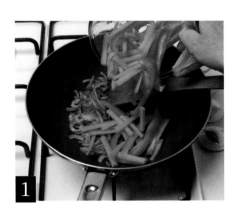

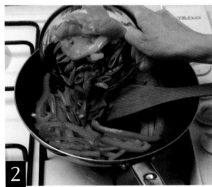

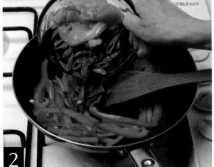

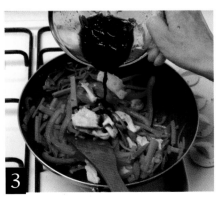

1 Heat the oil in a wok or large frying pan and cook the onion over a moderate heat until softened. Add the red pepper and carrot and stir-fry for 2–3 minutes.

2 Add the chicken strips and sugar snaps and cook, stirring, until the chicken is cooked through. This should take about 4–5 minutes.

3 Mix the sliced stem ginger with the syrup in a mixing bowl. Finely grate the zest from the lemon and squeeze the juice. Add to the stem ginger and mix. Stir in the soy sauce. Add this mixture to the wok and cook, stirring, for 2 minutes. Remove from the heat and serve with brown rice.

# Seeded Chicken Nuggets

*Family Favourite*

Chicken nuggets are even better when they are homemade, especially with the health benefits you get from linseeds and sesame seeds. Look out for oil pumps. They are very handy, giving a light spray of oil to your cooking without any fuss or mess.

### Serves 2

75g/3oz stale brown bread
3 tbsp sesame seeds
3 tbsp linseeds
2 skinless, boneless chicken
   breasts
2 tbsp wholemeal flour
1 egg
olive oil for spraying
salad and tomato ketchup
   to serve

### Serves 4

175g/6oz stale brown bread
6 tbsp sesame seeds
6 tbsp linseeds
4 skinless, boneless chicken
   breasts
4 tbsp wholemeal flour
2 eggs
olive oil for spraying
salad and tomato ketchup
   to serve

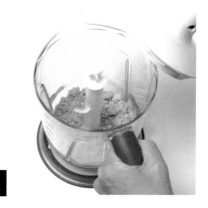

1 Preheat the oven to 200°C/400°F/Gas Mark 6. To make the breadcrumbs, remove the crusts from the bread and discard. Cut the bread into rough chunks and process in a blender or food processor until reduced to breadcrumbs. Tip onto a plate, add the seeds, mix and set to one side.

2 Slice the chicken breasts into bite-size chunks and set to one side. Place the flour on a plate. Beat the egg and pour into a shallow bowl.

3 Lightly oil a heavy-gauge baking sheet with a little

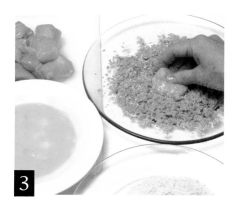

olive oil. Taking one piece of chicken at a time, dip it first in the flour then in the beaten egg, turning to coat. Finally dip it in the breadcrumbs, pressing firmly to make sure it is evenly coated. Place on the baking sheet and repeat the procedure with the remaining chicken.

4 Lightly spray the chicken pieces with olive oil. Bake in the preheated oven for 15–20 minutes, turning once halfway through.

5 Serve with salad and a little tomato ketchup for dipping.

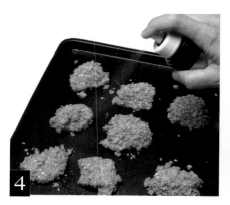

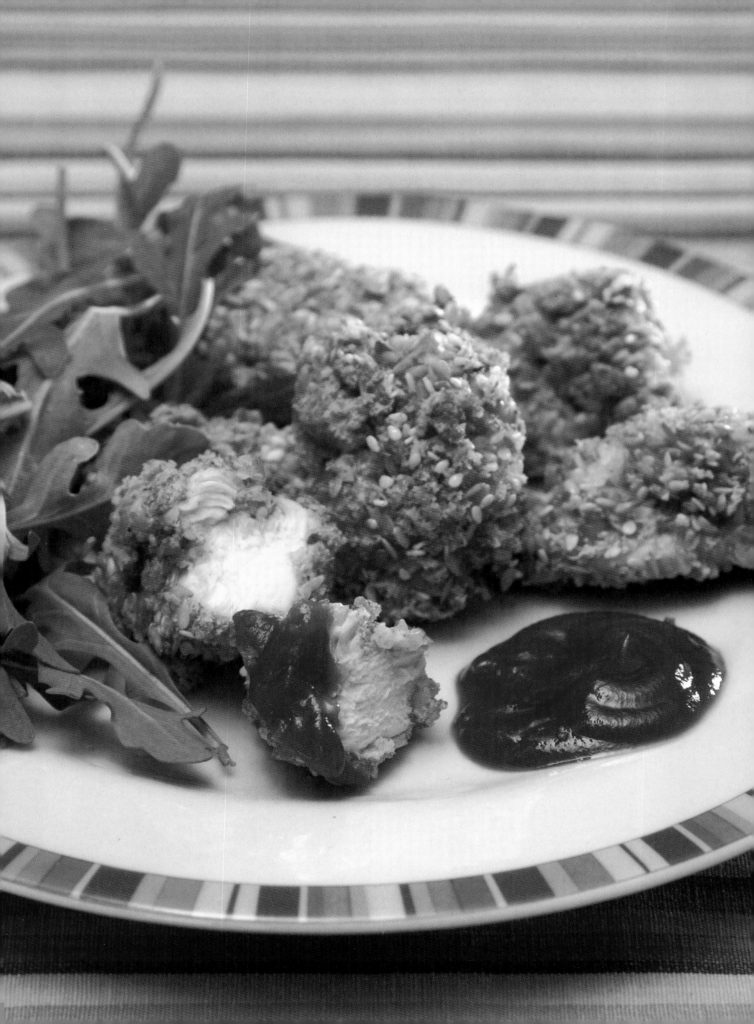

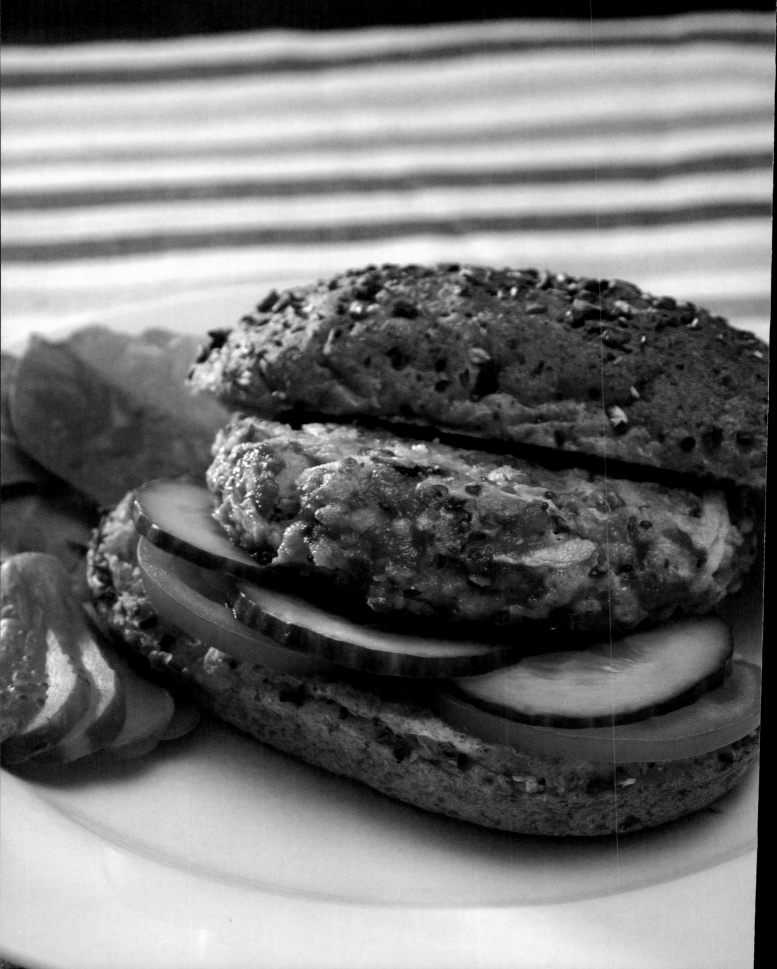

# Turkey & Apple Burgers

*Children's Choice*

These healthy burgers are quick and easy to make.

## Serves 2

40g/1½oz wholemeal bread,
  crusts removed
250g/9oz turkey mince
½ tbsp wholegrain mustard
1 small eating apple
½ egg, beaten
sunflower oil for spraying
2 burger buns
salad to serve

## Serves 4

75g/3oz wholemeal bread,
  crusts removed
500g/1lb 2oz turkey mince
1 tbsp wholegrain mustard
1 eating apple
1 egg, beaten
sunflower oil for spraying
4 burger buns
salad to serve

1 Roughly chop the bread and process in a blender or food processor to form breadcrumbs.

2 Place the turkey mince in a mixing bowl. Add the wholegrain mustard and breadcrumbs and mix.

3 Core and peel the apple and grate coarsely. Add it to the turkey and mix again. Stir in the beaten egg.

4 Using slightly damp hands, divide the mixture into 2 (4) equal pieces and shape each one into a burger. Spray each burger with a little oil.

5 Preheat the grill to moderate and then cook the burgers for 10 minutes, turning halfway, until golden and cooked through. Serve in buns with salad.

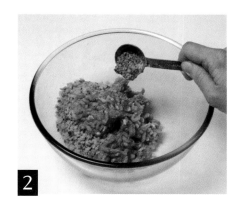

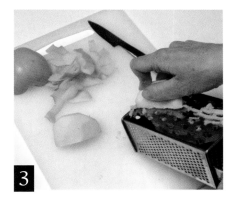

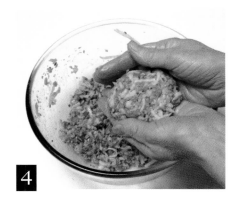

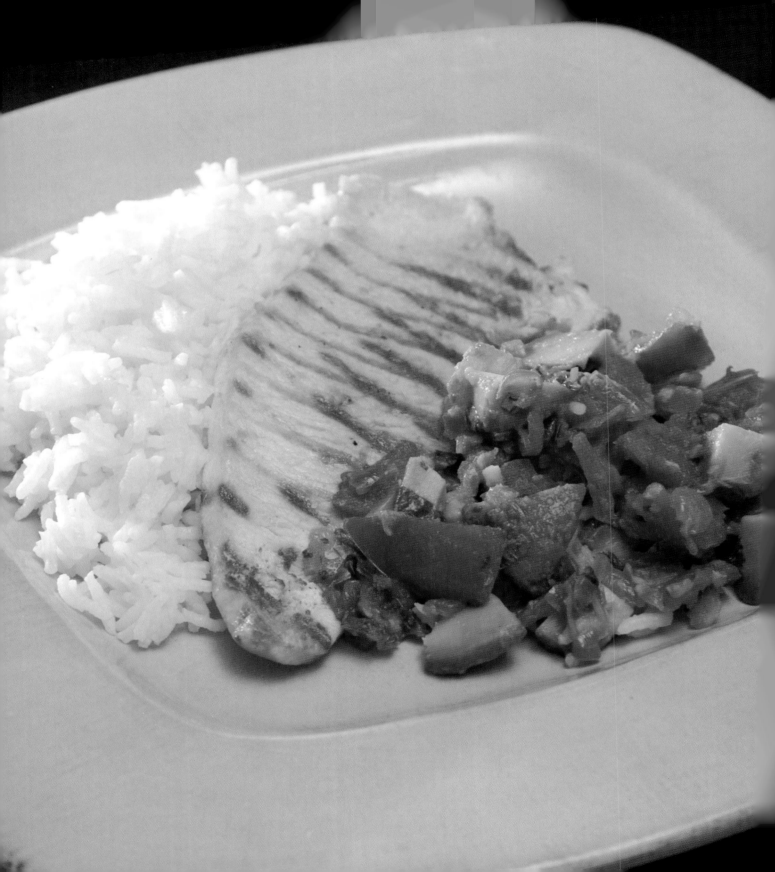

# Hot Guacamole with Turkey Steak

*Easy Entertaining*

Avocados are high in mono-unsaturated fats, which can be helpful in lowering cholesterol.

## Serves 2

½ tbsp olive oil
1 small red onion, finely
    chopped
1 small clove garlic, peeled
    and crushed
½ red chilli, chopped
2 tomatoes, deseeded and
    chopped
2 turkey steaks
1 small avocado
2 tbsp coriander, chopped
½ lime
basmati rice to serve

## Serves 4

1 tbsp olive oil
1 red onion, finely chopped
1 clove garlic, peeled and
    crushed
1 red chilli, chopped
4 tomatoes, deseeded and
    chopped
4 turkey steaks
1 avocado
4 tbsp fresh coriander,
    chopped
1 lime
basmati rice to serve

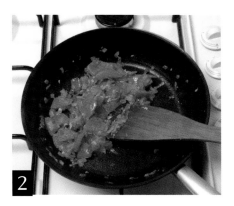

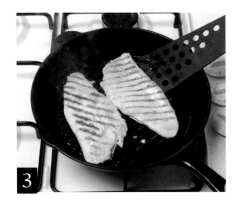

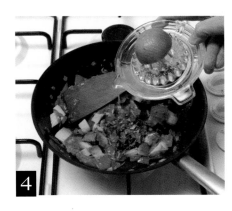

1 Heat the oil in a frying pan and cook the red onion until softened. Add the garlic and chilli and cook for 2–3 minutes, stirring.

2 Add the tomatoes and cook gently for about 10 minutes until they become softened and thick.

3 Heat a griddle over a moderately high heat and cook the turkey steaks for about 8 minutes, turning halfway, until piping hot and cooked through.

4 While the turkey is cooking, peel the avocado and chop the flesh. Add to the tomato mixture. Stir in the coriander and add the squeezed juice from the lime. Cook, stirring, for 3–4 minutes, until the mixture is piping hot.

5 Serve the turkey with some rice and a large spoonful of the hot guacamole.

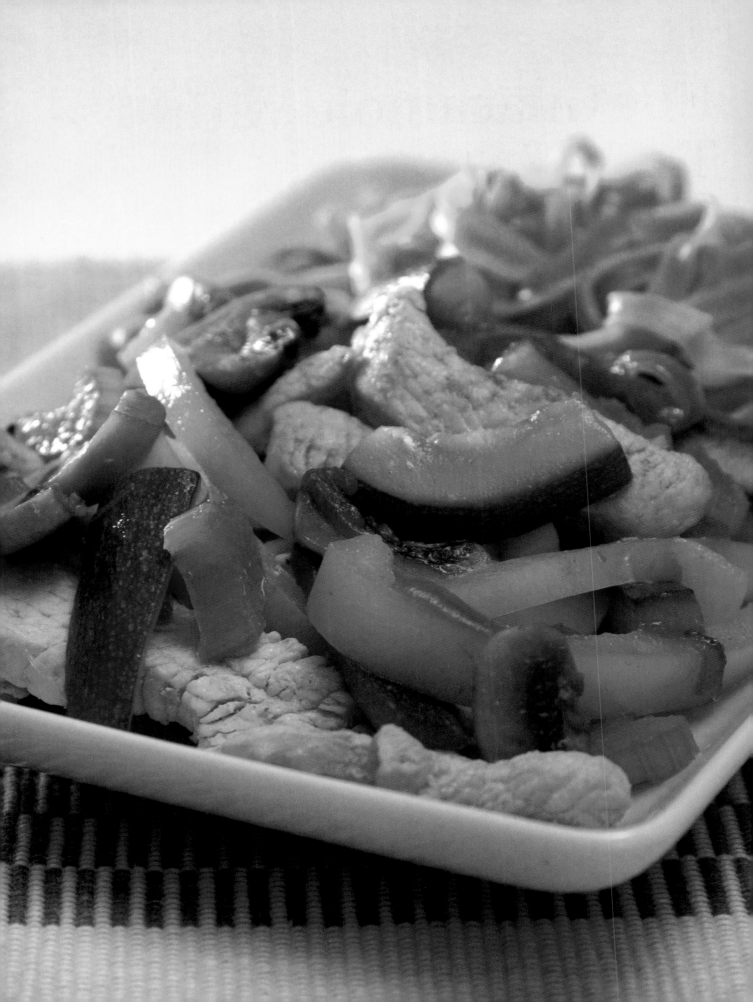

# Turkey Stir-fry

*One Pot*

Stir-fries are not only great because they are fast but because the quick cooking time preserves more of the nutrients.

## Serves 2

2 tsp olive oil
1 small red onion, peeled
and sliced
1 clove garlic, peeled and
crushed
2 sticks celery, sliced
200g/7oz turkey breast,
sliced into thin strips
1 small yellow pepper,
deseeded and thinly
sliced
1 courgette, trimmed and cut
into small batons
75g/3oz button mushrooms,
sliced
2 tbsp Worcestershire sauce
noodles or new potatoes
to serve

## Serves 4

4 tsp olive oil
1 red onion, peeled and
sliced
2 cloves garlic, peeled and
crushed
4 sticks celery, sliced
400g/14oz turkey breast,
sliced into thin strips
1 yellow pepper, deseeded
and thinly sliced
1 large courgette, trimmed
and cut into small batons
175g/6oz button mushrooms,
sliced
4 tbsp Worcestershire sauce
noodles or new potatoes to
serve

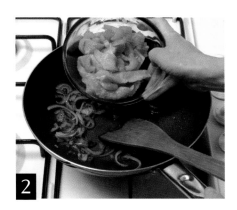

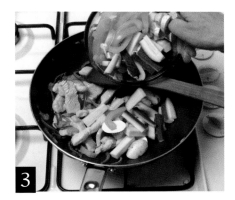

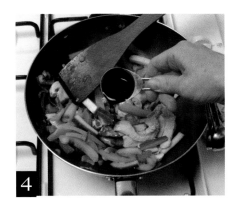

1 Heat the oil in a large wok over a high heat. Add the onion and stir-fry for 2–3 minutes.

2 Add the garlic, celery and turkey and continue to stir-fry for a further 2–3 minutes.

3 Add the pepper, courgette and mushrooms and cook, stirring, for 4–5 minutes or until

the pepper is just softened and piping hot.

4 Stir in the Worcestershire sauce and cook for 1 minute. Serve over noodles or accompanied by new potatoes.

# Pork Tenderloin Roast

*Family Favourite*

A tasty low-fat roast – perfect for Sunday lunch.

## Serves 2

**1 small pork tenderloin**
**½ tsp olive oil**
**1½ tbsp fresh rosemary,
    chopped**
**1½ tbsp fresh parsley,
    chopped**
**½ tbsp black peppercorns**
**1 tbsp crème fraîche**
**vegetables and new potatoes
    to serve**

## Serves 4

**1 large or 2 small pork
    tenderloins**
**1 tsp olive oil**
**3 tbsp fresh rosemary,
    chopped**
**3 tbsp fresh parsley,
    chopped**
**1 tbsp black peppercorns**
**2 tbsp crème fraîche**
**vegetables and new potatoes
    to serve**

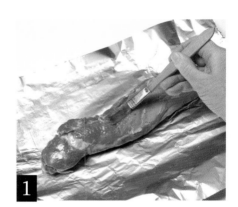

1 Preheat the oven to 190°C/375°F/Gas Mark 5. Brush a large sheet of tin foil with a little of the oil. Place the tenderloin in the centre of the foil. Using the remaining oil, brush the tenderloin all over.

2 In a bowl, mix together the chopped rosemary and parsley. Use a pestle and mortar to roughly crush the peppercorns and add them to the chopped herbs. Mix.

3 Press the herb and pepper mixture over the tenderloin to cover evenly. Pull the tin foil up over the meat to cover loosely and pinch the edges together to seal it. Place

in a roasting tin and cook in the preheated oven for 20 minutes per 450g/1lb plus 20 minutes.

4 Once the meat is cooked, remove it from the oven and leave in a warm place for 15 minutes for the meat to rest. At the end of this time, open the foil and pour any juices that have collected into a small saucepan. Stir in the crème fraîche and gently heat to almost boiling. Remove from the heat. Carve the meat into thin slices and serve with the crème fraîche sauce, vegetables and new potatoes.

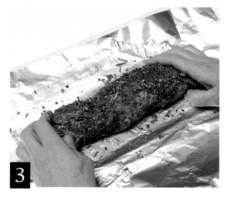

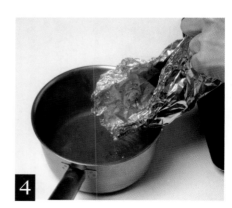

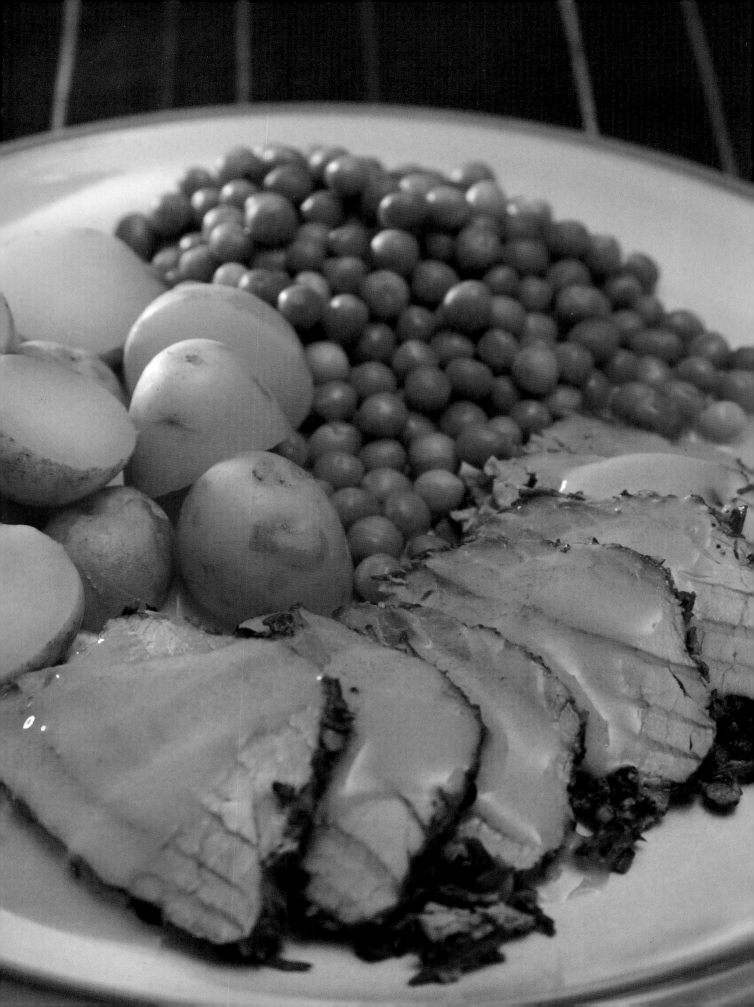

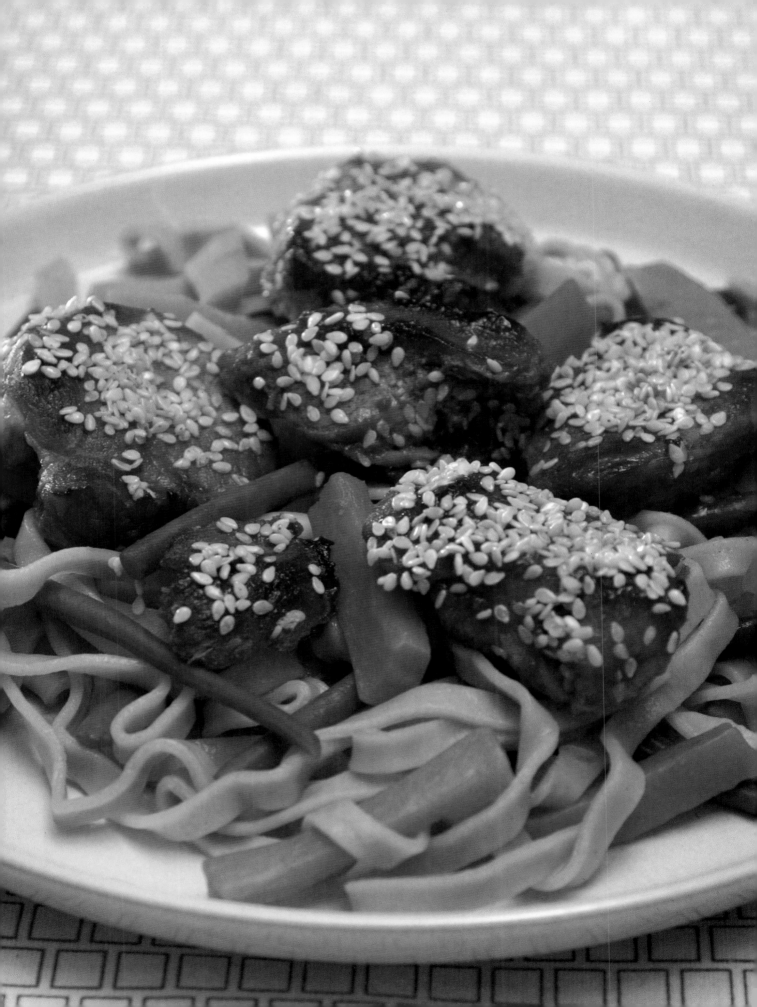

# Hoisin & Sesame Pork

*Easy Entertaining*

People often think of pork as being fatty, but if you get a nice lean cut it is almost as low in fat as skinless chicken.

### Serves 2

- 1 small pork tenderloin
- 2 tbsp hoisin sauce
- 1 tbsp rice vinegar
- 2.5cm/1in piece fresh ginger, peeled and finely grated
- 1 clove garlic, peeled and crushed
- ½ tsp sesame oil
- 100g/4oz green beans trimmed
- 100g/4oz carrots, peeled and cut into batons
- 2 tbsp sesame seeds
- noodles to serve

### Serves 4

- 2 small pork tenderloins
- 4 tbsp hoisin sauce
- 2 tbsp rice vinegar
- 5cm/2in piece fresh ginger, peeled and finely grated
- 2 cloves garlic, peeled and crushed
- 1 tsp sesame oil
- 200g/7oz green beans trimmed
- 200g/7oz carrots, peeled and cut into batons
- 4 tbsp sesame seeds
- noodles to serve

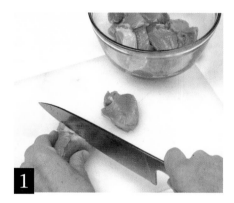

1 Using a sharp knife cut the tenderloin into thick slices and place in a glass or plastic mixing bowl.

2 Add the hoisin sauce, rice vinegar, ginger, garlic and sesame oil and mix thoroughly to coat the pork. Cover and chill for 2–6 hours.

3 Preheat the grill to moderately high. Pour the pork and marinade into a small roasting tin and cook for 8–10 minutes, turning halfway, until cooked through.

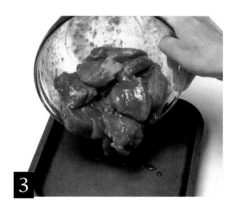

4 Bring a saucepan of water to the boil. Add the beans and carrots and cook for 3–4 minutes. Drain and keep warm.

5 Sprinkle the sesame seeds over the pork and grill for a further 1–2 minutes, or until the sesame seeds become golden. Serve with the carrots, beans and noodles.

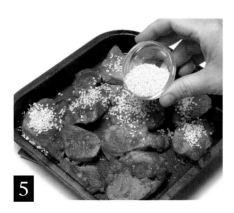

# Chilli

*Family Favourite*

Generally chilli is made with beef but in this recipe pork, which is lower in fat, is used.

## Serves 2

225g/8oz lean pork, diced
½ tsp paprika
½ tsp ground cumin
½ tsp oregano
¼ tsp chilli powder, or
   according to taste
1 tsp olive oil
1 small onion, peeled and
   chopped
1 small clove garlic, peeled
   and crushed
1 x 200g/7oz can tomatoes,
   chopped
1 carrot, peeled
1 courgette, trimmed
1 tbsp tomato purée
1 x 200g/7oz can red kidney
   beans, rinsed and drained
brown rice and low-fat
  yoghurt to serve

## Serves 4

450g/1lb lean pork, diced
1tsp paprika
1 tsp ground cumin
1 tsp oregano
½ tsp chilli powder, or
   according to taste
2 tsp olive oil
1 onion, peeled and chopped
1 clove garlic, peeled and
   crushed
1 x 400g/14oz can tomatoes,
   chopped
1 large carrot, peeled
1 large courgette, trimmed
2 tbsp tomato purée
1 x 400g/14oz can red kidney
   beans, rinsed and
   drained
brown rice and low-fat
   yoghurt to serve

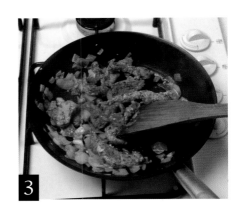

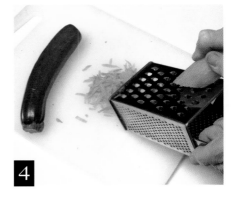

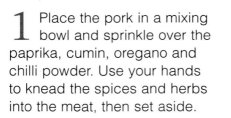

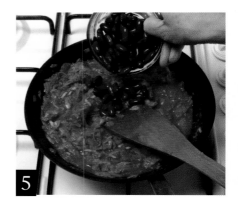

1 Place the pork in a mixing bowl and sprinkle over the paprika, cumin, oregano and chilli powder. Use your hands to knead the spices and herbs into the meat, then set aside.

2 Heat the oil in a large frying pan and cook the onion and garlic over a moderate heat until softened.

3 Add the meat and cook, stirring, until browned on all sides. Add the tomatoes and bring gently to the boil.

4 Coarsely grate the carrot and courgette and add to the pan, stirring well to mix. Stir in the tomato purée and bring gently to the boil. Reduce the heat to a simmer and cook, uncovered, for 15 minutes.

5 Stir in the kidney beans and continue to cook for a further 15 minutes. Serve with brown rice and a little low-fat yoghurt if desired.

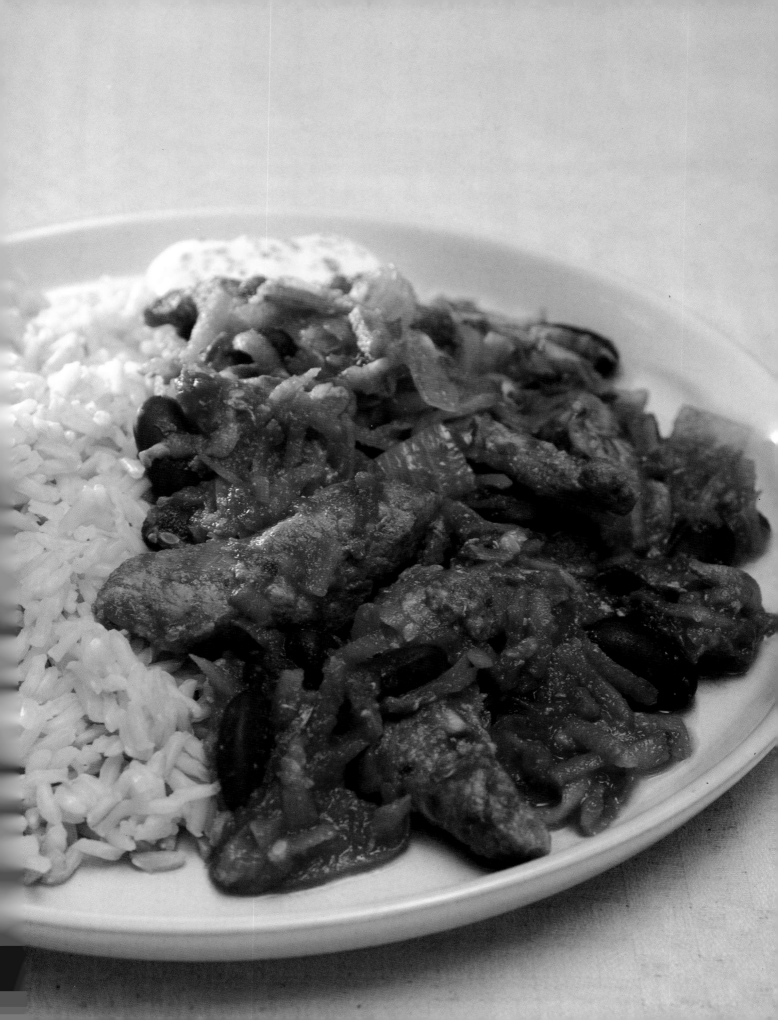

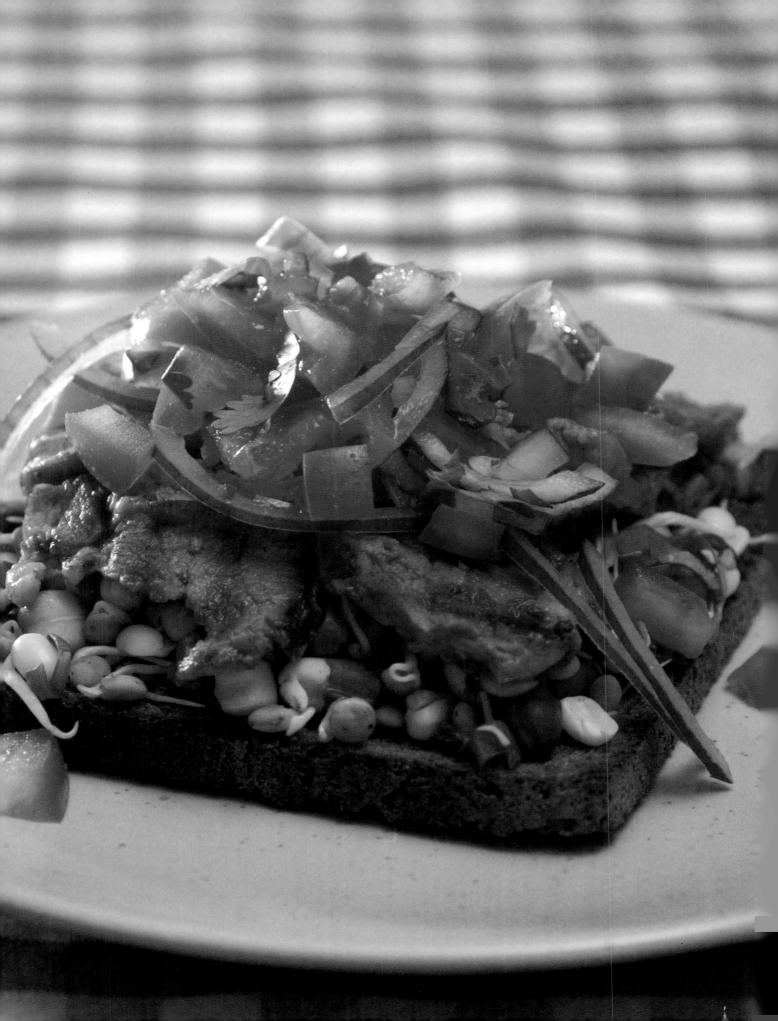

# Lamb & Salsa Open Sandwich

*Quick and Easy*

Look for lean lamb and trim as much fat as you can before cooking. Cooking on a griddle pan will allow the fat to drain away from the meat as it cooks.

### Serves 2

**2 tomatoes**
**½ green chilli**
**½ small red onion**
**½ lime**
**1 tsp caster sugar**
**3 tbsp fresh coriander, chopped**
**1 small clove garlic**
**200g/7oz lamb neck fillets**
**2 thick slices wholemeal or granary bread**
**100g/4oz mixed sprouted beans**

### Serves 4

**4 tomatoes**
**1 green chilli**
**1 small red onion**
**1 lime**
**2 tsp caster sugar**
**6 tbsp fresh coriander, chopped**
**1 clove garlic**
**400g/14oz lamb neck fillets**
**4 thick slices wholemeal or granary bread**
**200g/7oz mixed sprouted beans**

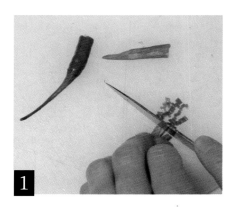

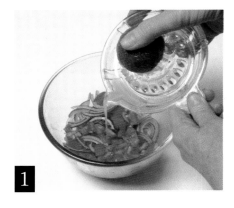

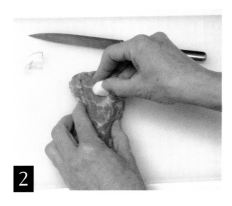

1 Deseed and chop the tomatoes and place in a mixing bowl. Finely chop the chilli, removing the seeds if you prefer less heat in your chilli. Add to the tomato. Peel and finely slice the red onion and add to the mixing bowl. Squeeze the juice from the lime and pour over the tomato mixture. Add the caster sugar and toss well to mix. Sprinkle over the coriander and set to one side.

2 Cut the garlic in half, rub the cut side over the lamb and then discard. Heat a griddle pan over a moderately high heat and cook the lamb for 8–10 minutes, turning until evenly browned all over. Remove from the pan and place on a chopping board. Using a sharp knife, slice thinly.

3 Toast the bread and place on serving plates. Divide the sprouted beans between the toast, top with the sliced lamb, followed by a large spoonful of the tomato salsa. Serve.

# Thai Beef Salad

*Easy Entertaining*

A light salad with thin strips of sirloin steak and a hot, sweet, sour dressing.

### Serves 2

¼ cucumber
4 radishes, trimmed
2 spring onions
1 carrot, peeled
1 tbsp fresh lime juice
1 tbsp nam pla
1 tsp sugar
½ red chilli
1 clove garlic, peeled
250g/9oz sirloin steak
1 tbsp fresh mint leaves
4 tbsp fresh coriander leaves

### Serves 4

½ cucumber
8 radishes, trimmed
4 spring onions
2 carrots, peeled
2 tbsp fresh lime juice
2 tbsp nam pla
2 tsp sugar
1 red chilli
2 cloves garlic, peeled
450g/1lb sirloin steak
2 tbsp fresh mint leaves
8 tbsp fresh coriander leaves

1 Deseed the cucumber, thinly slice and place in a mixing bowl. Finely slice the radishes and spring onions and add to the cucumber.

2 Using a vegetable peeler, cut the carrot into thin strips and stir into the cucumber mixture.

3 In a small non-metallic bowl, mix the lime juice with the nam pla, sugar and chilli. Set to one side.

4 Heat a griddle pan over a high heat. Rub the steak with the cut side of the garlic and then discard. Cook the steak in the preheated pan for approximately 3–4 minutes each side. If you prefer your steak well done cook for a further 1–2 minutes until cooked to your taste.

5 Remove from the heat and place the steak on a chopping board. Cut into thin strips with a sharp knife.

6 Divide the salad between the serving plates. Top with strips of the beef. Drizzle over the lime juice mixture and scatter with the mint and coriander leaves. Serve.

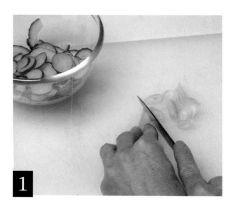

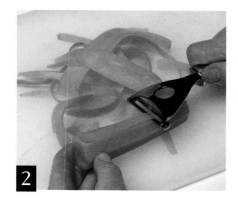

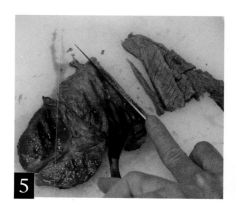

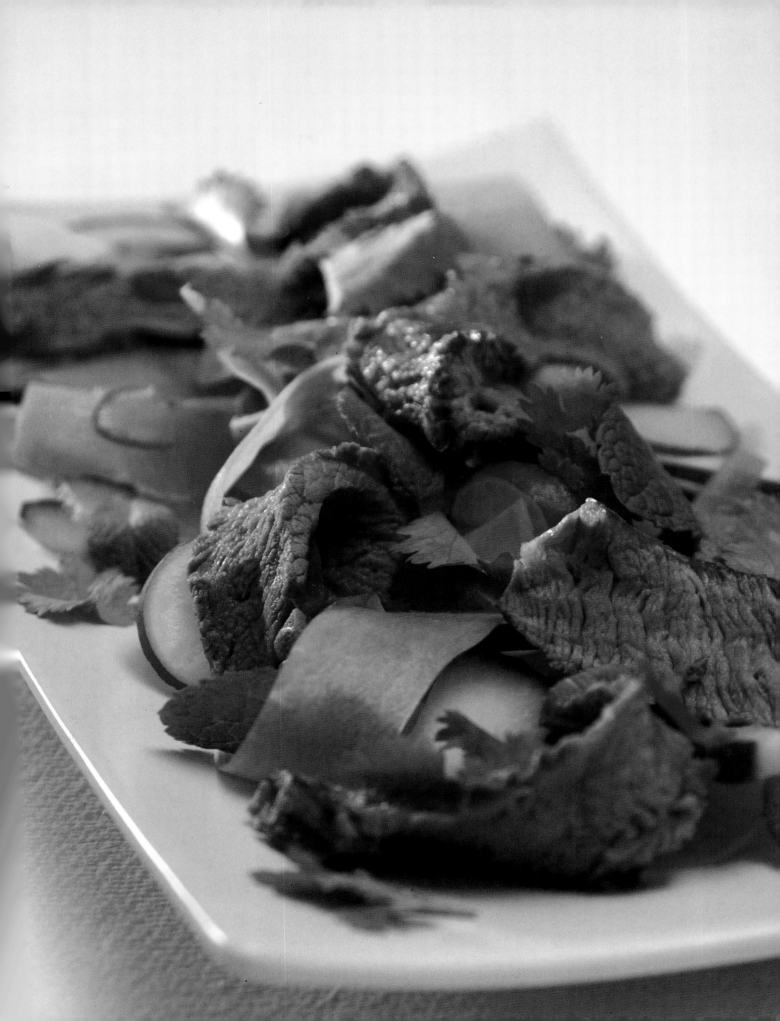

# Light-curried Prawns

*One Pot*

Curries are often high in fat. This recipe shows that you can still have all the flavour without the high fat.

## Serves 2

½ tbsp oil
½ onion, finely chopped
½ tsp ground cumin
¼ tsp chilli powder
225g/8oz tomatoes, skinned and chopped
½ tbsp ground almonds
125g/4½oz frozen prawns, defrosted
75ml/2½fl oz natural yoghurt
2 tbsp fresh coriander, chopped

## Serves 4

1 tbsp oil
1 medium onion, finely chopped
1 tsp ground cumin
½ tsp chilli powder
450g/1lb tomatoes, skinned and chopped
1 tbsp ground almonds
250g/9oz frozen prawns, defrosted
150ml/¼pt natural yoghurt
4 tbsp fresh coriander, chopped

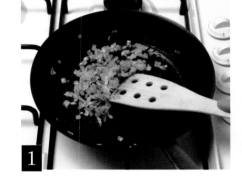

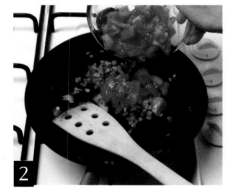

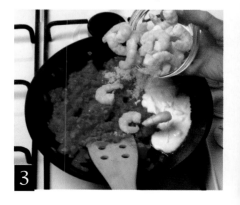

1 Heat the oil in a large frying pan. Add the onion and cook over a moderate heat, stirring from time to time, until they start to turn golden.

2 Add the spices and cook for 1 minute before adding the tomatoes. Cook for 5 minutes, or until the mixture thickens.

3 Add the almonds, prawns and yoghurt and cook for a further 5 minutes until piping hot. Stir through the chopped coriander and serve with basmati rice.

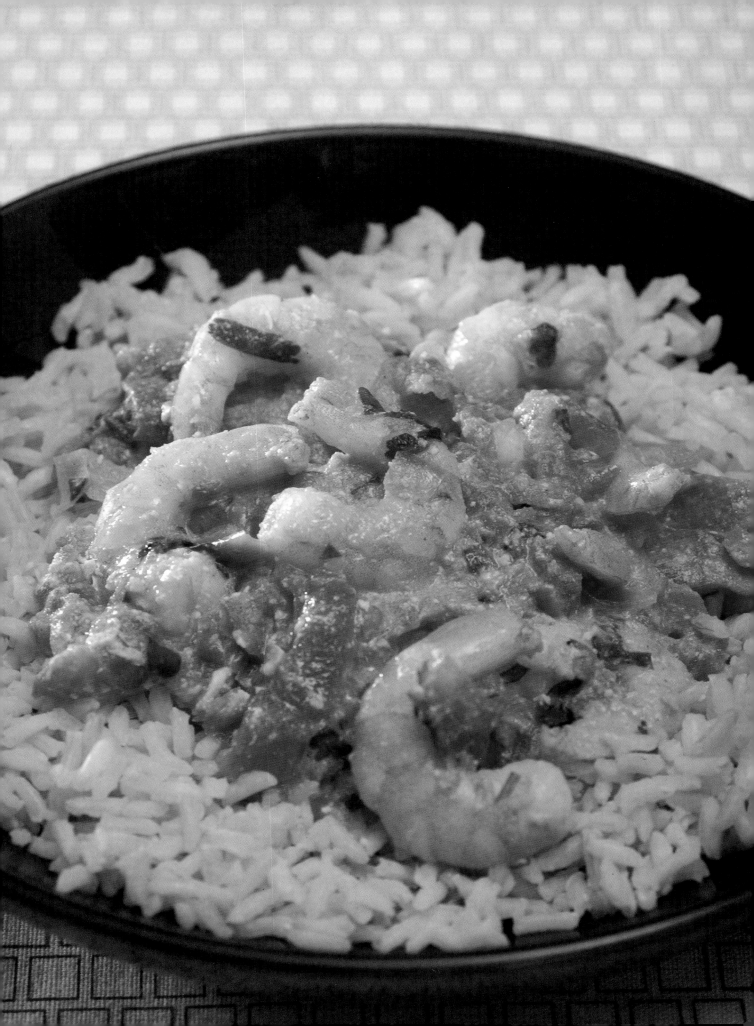

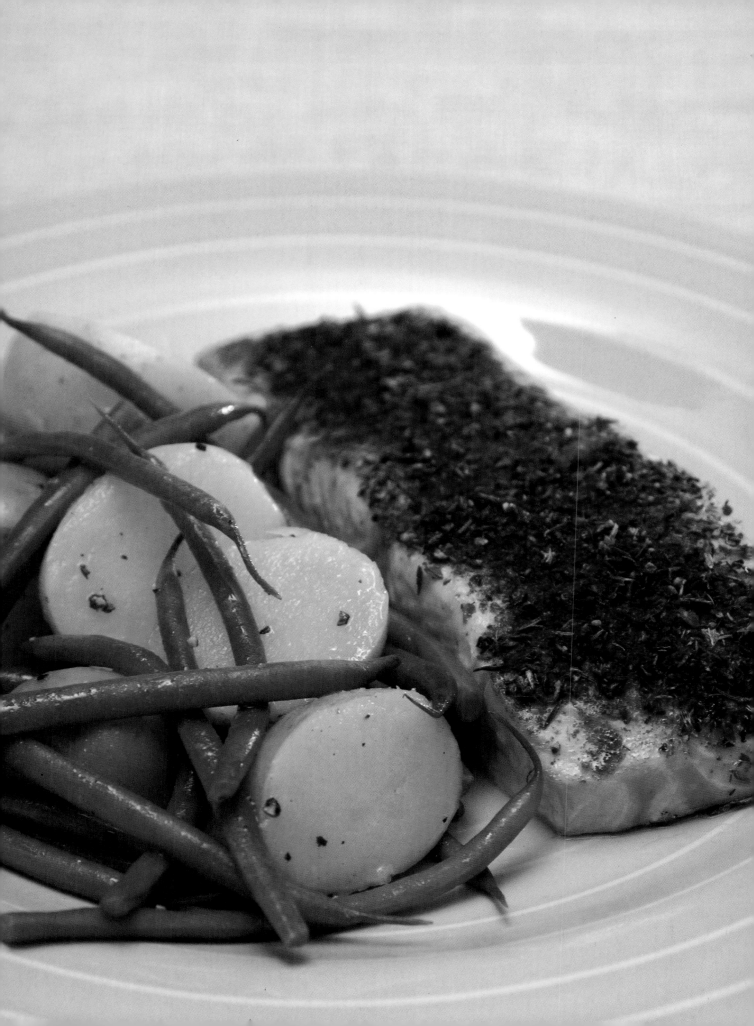

# Spiced Salmon Steaks

*Easy Entertaining*

Salmon is a very versatile fish and a good source of protein and vitamins A, B12 and D, plus the all-important omega-3 fatty acids.

## Serves 2

- **1 tsp paprika**
- **¼ tsp chilli powder**
- **¼ tsp black pepper**
- **¼ tsp oregano**
- **¼ tsp dried basil**
- **¼ tsp dried thyme**
- **2 x 175g/6oz salmon steaks**
- **2 tsp olive oil, plus a little for spraying**
- **1 tbsp lemon juice**
- **½ tsp Dijon mustard**
- **black pepper to taste**
- **250g/9oz new potatoes, cleaned and halved if large**
- **150g/5oz fine beans, trimmed**

## Serves 4

- **2 tsp paprika**
- **½ tsp chilli powder**
- **½ tsp black pepper**
- **½ tsp oregano**
- **½ tsp dried basil**
- **½ tsp dried thyme**
- **4 x 175g/6oz salmon steaks**
- **4 tsp olive oil, plus a little for spraying**
- **2 tbsp lemon juice**
- **1 tsp Dijon mustard**
- **black pepper to taste**
- **500g/1lb 2oz new potatoes, cleaned and halved if large**
- **300g/10½oz fine beans, trimmed**

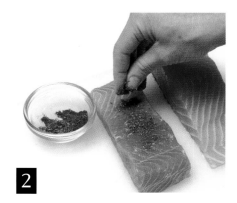

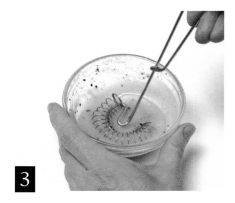

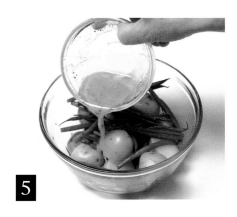

1 Preheat the oven to 200°C/400°F/Gas Mark 6. Place a heavy-gauge baking tray in the oven to heat. Mix the paprika, chilli powder, black pepper, oregano, basil and thyme in a small mixing bowl.

2 Rub the spice mixture into the fish to coat. Spray with a little oil. Set to one side in a cool place.

3 In a small mixing bowl whisk the oil with the lemon juice, mustard and black pepper. Bring a saucepan of water to the boil and cook the new potatoes for 10–12 minutes until tender. Add the green beans for last 3–4 minutes. Check that the vegetables are tender before draining, and cook for a few minutes more if necessary.

4 While the potatoes are cooking, place the steaks on the preheated baking tray and bake for 10–12 minutes until hot and cooked through.

5 Toss the lemon and olive oil mixture through the drained potatoes and beans. Serve with the salmon steaks.

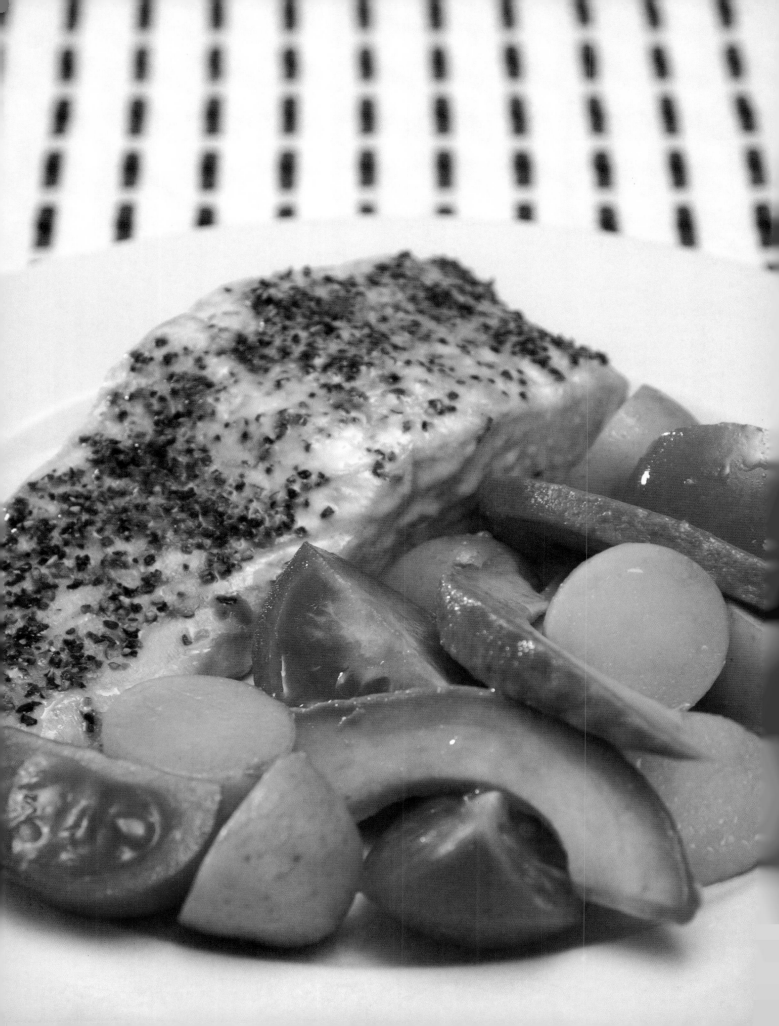

# Lemon & Black Pepper Salmon with Avocado Salad

*Easy Entertaining*

Avocados are highly calorific but also very good for us. So enjoy them but not too often!

### Serves 2

**1 tsp black peppercorns, crushed**
**¼ tsp lemon zest**
**2 x 175g/6oz salmon fillets**
**150g/5oz small new potatoes**
**4 small ripe tomatoes, quartered**
**1 medium avocado**
**½ tbsp balsamic vinegar**
**1 tbsp olive oil**

### Serves 4

**2 tsp black peppercorns, crushed**
**½ tsp lemon zest**
**4 x 175g/6oz salmon fillets**
**275g/10oz small new potatoes**
**8 small ripe tomatoes, quartered**
**2 medium avocados**
**1 tbsp balsamic vinegar**
**2 tbsp olive oil**

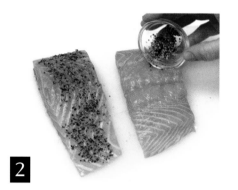

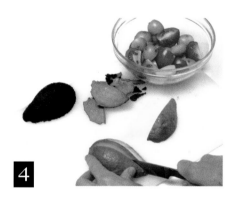

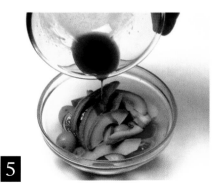

1 Preheat the oven to 200°C/400°F/Gas Mark 6 and place a heavy-gauge baking tray in the oven to heat.

2 Mix the crushed black peppercorns and lemon together. Divide equally between the salmon pieces, pressing the mixture into the flesh. Place the salmon on the preheated baking tray and cook for 8–10 minutes.

3 While the salmon is cooking, bring a saucepan of water to the boil and cook the potatoes until tender. Drain and place in a mixing bowl.

4 Add the tomatoes to the warm potatoes. Peel and slice the avocado(s). Mix into the potatoes and tomatoes.

5 Whisk the balsamic vinegar and olive oil together and drizzle over the potato mixture. Divide the avocado salad between the serving plates and place a salmon fillet on each. Serve.

# Sesame-crusted Salmon

*Easy Entertaining*

Salmon is an excellent source of protein and it also falls into the category of an "oily fish", which means it can be useful in guarding against heart disease if eaten on a regular basis.

## Serves 2

- 1 tbsp sesame seeds
- 1 tbsp sunflower seeds
- 1 tbsp cornflour
- 1 tbsp soy sauce
- 2 tbsp rice wine vinegar
- 2 tsp honey
- ½ tsp sesame oil
- 1 small clove garlic, peeled and crushed
- 1cm/½in fresh ginger, peeled and finely grated
- 175g/6oz carrots, peeled
- 225g/8oz broccoli
- 2 tsp sunflower oil
- 2 large shallots, peeled and sliced
- 2 x 175g/6oz salmon fillets, skinned and cut into strips

## Serves 4

- 2 tbsp sesame seeds
- 2 tbsp sunflower seeds
- 2 tbsp cornflour
- 2 tbsp soy sauce
- 4 tbsp rice wine vinegar
- 4 tsp honey
- 1 tsp sesame oil
- 1 clove garlic, peeled and crushed
- 2.5cm/1in fresh ginger, peeled and finely grated
- 350g/12oz carrots, peeled
- 450g/1lb broccoli
- 4 tsp sunflower oil
- 4 large shallots, peeled and sliced
- 4 x 175g/6oz salmon fillets, skinned and cut into strips

1 Toast the seeds in a non-stick frying pan over a moderate heat.

2 Mix the cornflour and soy sauce to form a smooth paste. Add the vinegar, honey, sesame oil, garlic and ginger. Mix and set to one side.

3 Cut the carrots into batons. Break the broccoli into florets and cut the thick part of the stem into thin slices.

4 Heat the sunflower oil in a wok. Cook the shallots over a high heat until soft. Add the carrots and broccoli. Stir-fry for 2–3 minutes. Remove from the pan and keep warm.

5 Add the salmon to the wok. Cook for 2–3 minutes over a high heat. Pour over the cornflour mix. Stir gently until it thickens. To serve, spoon the salmon over the vegetables and sprinkle with seeds.

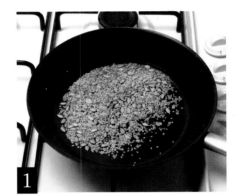

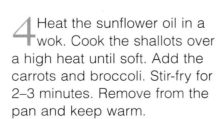

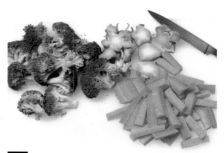

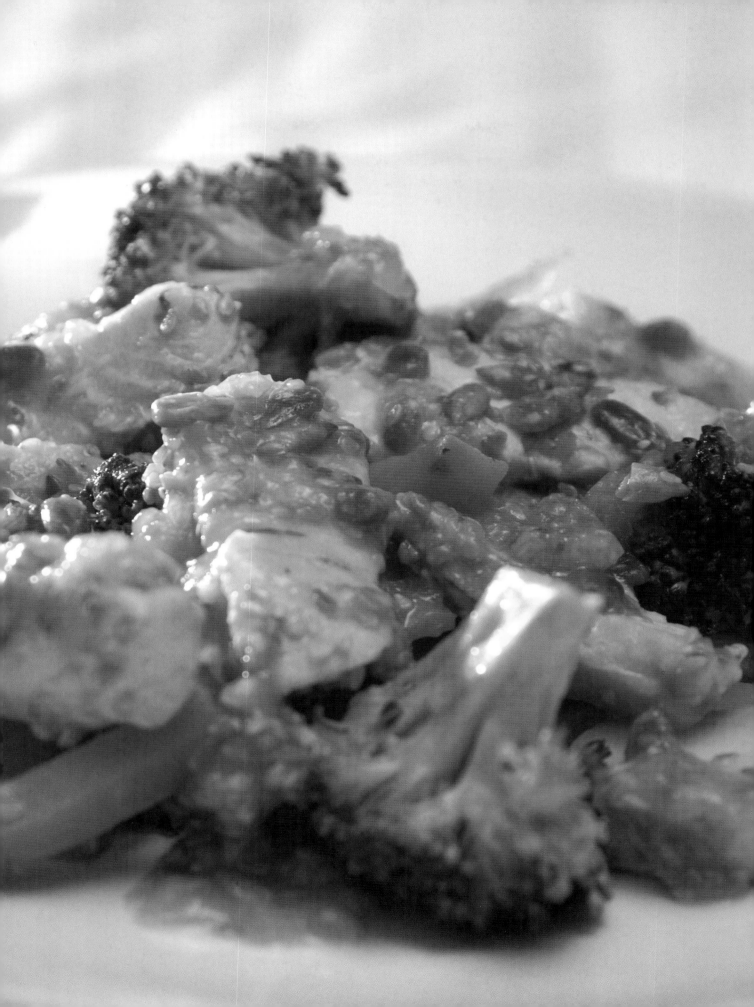

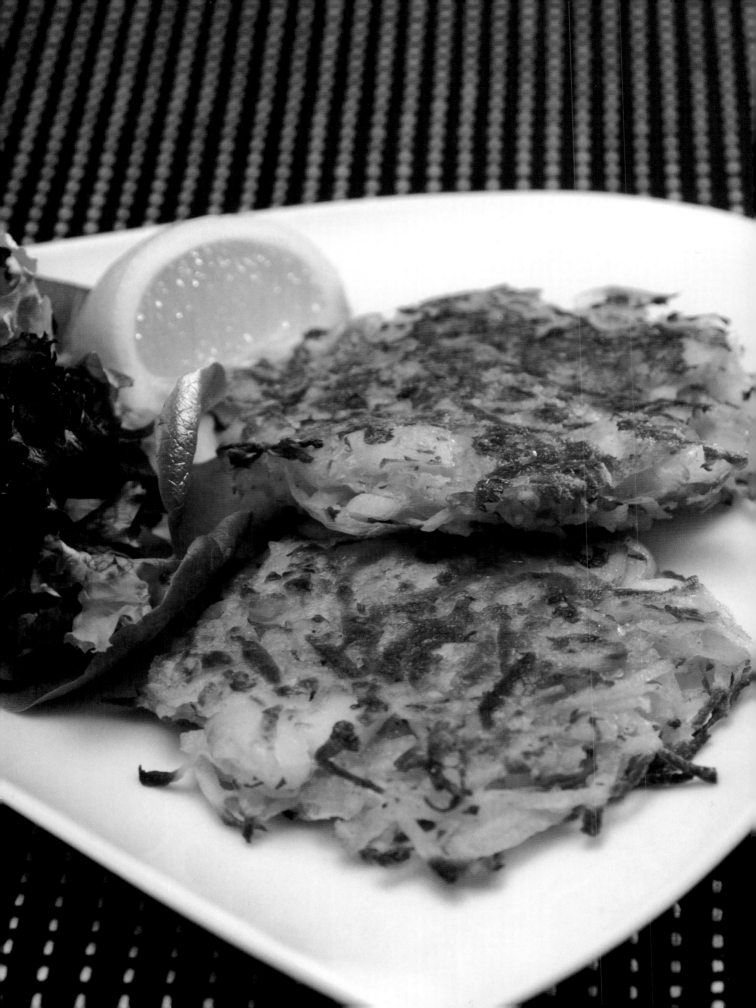

# Smoked Haddock Fish Cakes

*Family Favourite*

Baking these fish cakes instead of frying them reduces their fat content considerably.

## Serves 2

**200g/7oz smoked haddock**
**300g/10½oz waxy potatoes,**
   **peeled**
**1 small onion, peeled**
**1 tbsp fresh parsley,**
   **chopped**
**1 tbsp olive oil**
**1 tsp mild curry powder**
**steamed vegetables or salad**
   **and lemon wedges to**
   **serve**

## Serves 4

**400g/14oz smoked haddock**
**600g/1lb 5oz waxy potatoes,**
   **peeled**
**1 onion, peeled**
**2 tbsp fresh parsley,**
   **chopped**
**2 tbsp olive oil**
**2 tsp mild curry powder**
**steamed vegetables or salad**
   **and lemon wedges to**
   **serve**

1 Preheat the oven to 200°C/400°F/Gas Mark 6. Place the haddock in a shallow dish. Pour over enough boiling water to cover the fish and set to one side for 10 minutes. Remove the fish from the water, pull away the skin and discard. Flake the fish into a large mixing bowl, checking for bones as you do so.

2 Coarsely grate the potatoes and onion. Pat dry with a clean tea towel or kitchen paper. Add to the fish with the parsley and toss lightly to mix.

3 Mix the olive oil with the curry powder and drizzle it over the fish and potato mixture, gently tossing to mix.

4 Divide the mixture into 4 (8) and roughly shape into rounds. Place on a heavy-gauge baking sheet and bake in the preheated oven for 20–25 minutes, turning halfway through. Serve with the lemon wedges for squeezing.

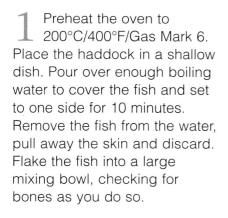

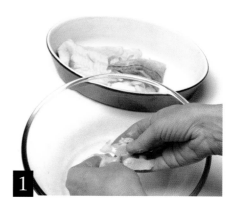

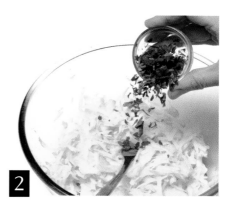

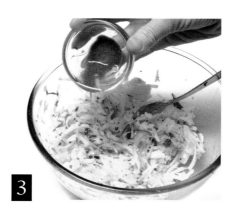

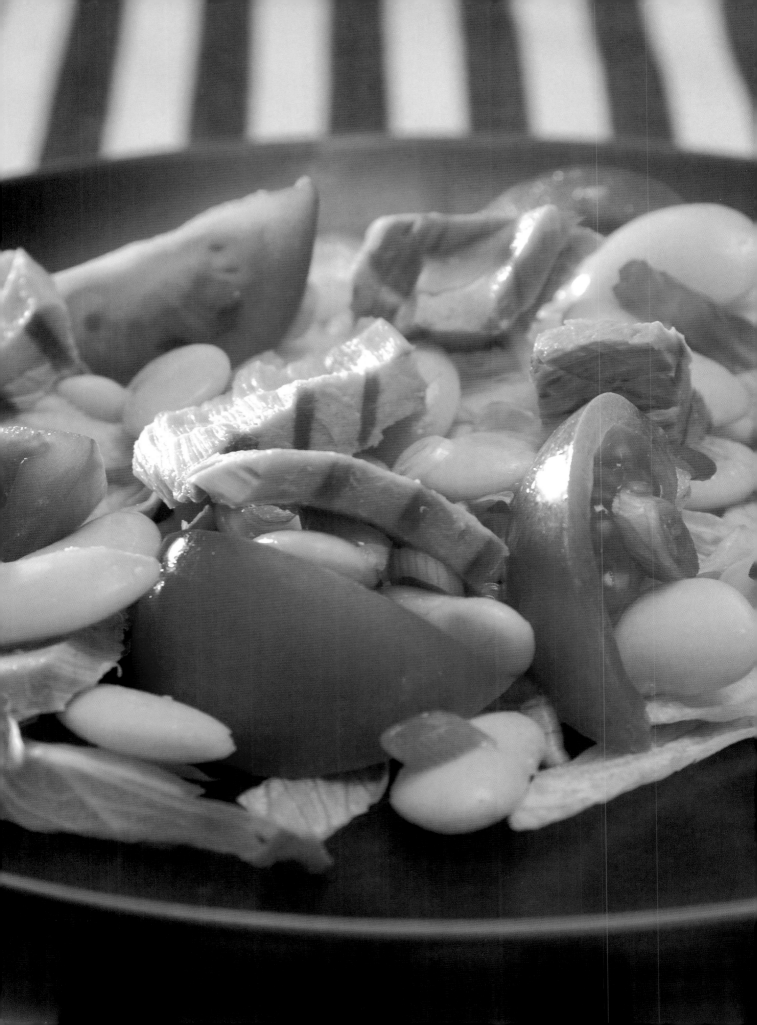

# Tuna & White Bean Salad

*Quick and Easy*

Perfect for a summer picnic, this is a tasty, protein-packed salad.

### Serves 2

- **175g/6oz fresh tuna steak**
- **1 tbsp olive oil**
- **2 tsp cider vinegar**
- **1 small clove garlic, peeled**
- **¼ tsp sea salt**
- **1 x 200g/7oz can butter beans**
- **3 small ripe tomatoes, quartered**
- **2 spring onions, trimmed and finely sliced**
- **100g/4oz crisp lettuce, shredded**

### Serves 4

- **350g/12oz fresh tuna steak**
- **2 tbsp olive oil**
- **4 tsp cider vinegar**
- **1 clove garlic, peeled**
- **½ tsp sea salt**
- **1 x 400g/14oz can butter beans**
- **6 small ripe tomatoes, quartered**
- **4 spring onions, trimmed and finely sliced**
- **200g/7oz crisp lettuce, shredded**

1 Preheat a griddle pan over a moderate heat and cook the tuna for about 8 minutes, turning halfway through. The cooking time depends on the thickness of the tuna – it should be piping hot and flake easily when tested with a fork. Set to one side.

2 Place the olive oil and cider vinegar in a small mixing bowl and, using a fork or small whisk, mix thoroughly. Use a mortar and pestle to crush the clove of peeled garlic with the salt until it forms a paste. Stir the garlic paste into the oil and vinegar and whisk again.

3 Place the beans, quartered tomatoes, sliced spring onions and shredded lettuce in a serving bowl. Drizzle over the oil and vinegar dressing and toss to mix.

4 Flake the tuna over the salad and toss gently, ensuring you don't break the fish up too much. Serve.

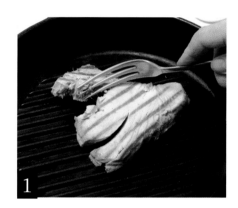

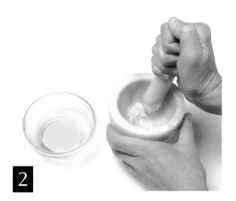

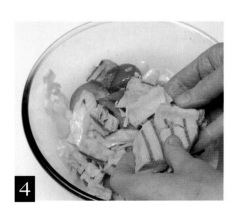

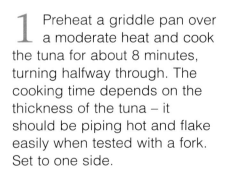

# Warm Tuna & Roasted Pepper Salad

*Easy Entertaining*

Fresh tuna is rich in omega-3 fatty acids, which have numerous health benefits.

## Serves 2

**1½ mixed sweet peppers**
**1 tbsp olive oil**
**300g/10½ oz new potatoes**
**1 tsp red wine vinegar**
**1 tsp wholegrain mustard**
**2 x 150g/5oz tuna steaks**

## Serves 4

**3 mixed sweet peppers**
**2 tbsp olive oil**
**600g/1lb 5oz new potatoes**
**2 tsp red wine vinegar**
**2 tsp wholegrain mustard**
**4 x 150g/5oz tuna steaks**

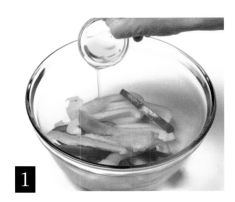

1 Preheat the oven to 200°C/400°F/Gas Mark 6. Halve the peppers, deseed and cut into slices. Place the sliced peppers in a mixing bowl, drizzle over a third of the olive oil and toss well to coat.

2 Spread the peppers in a single layer over a large baking tray and cook in the preheated oven for 25 minutes, turning them once halfway through.

3 Bring a large pan of water to the boil and cook the new potatoes for approximately 10 minutes until they are tender. Drain and set aside.

4 Whisk the remaining oil with the vinegar in a small mixing bowl. Add the mustard and whisk again.

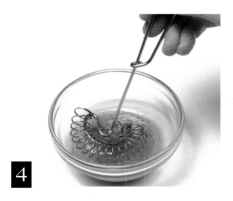

5 Preheat a griddle pan over a moderately high heat and cook the tuna steaks for about 4–5 minutes each side, until piping hot. Remove from the heat.

6 To serve, mix the roasted pepper strips with the new potatoes and drizzle over the mustard dressing. Roughly flake the tuna and add to the potatoes and peppers. Toss lightly to mix and divide between the serving plates while still warm.

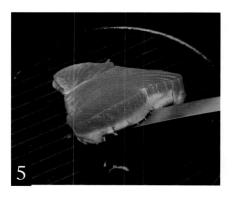

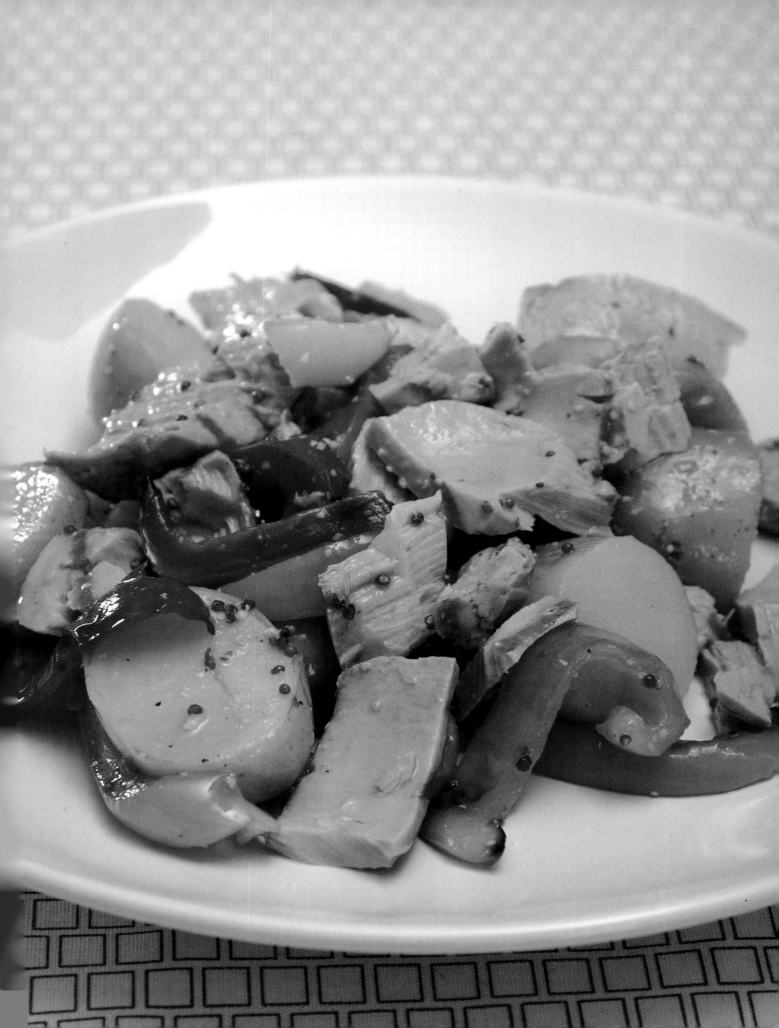

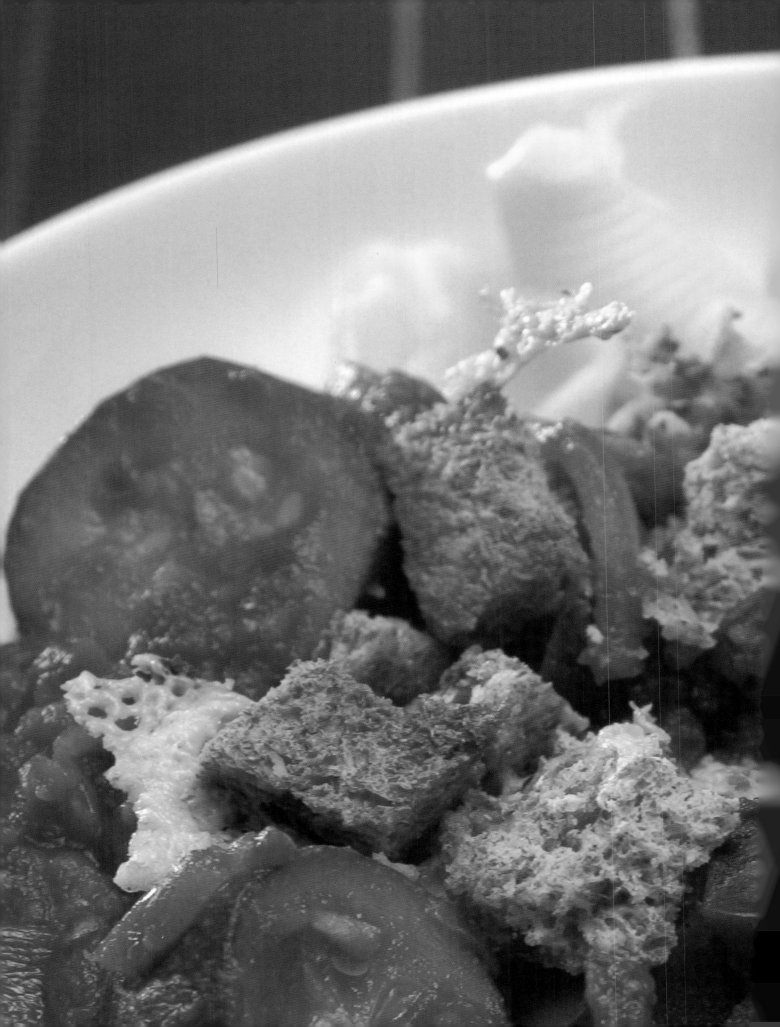

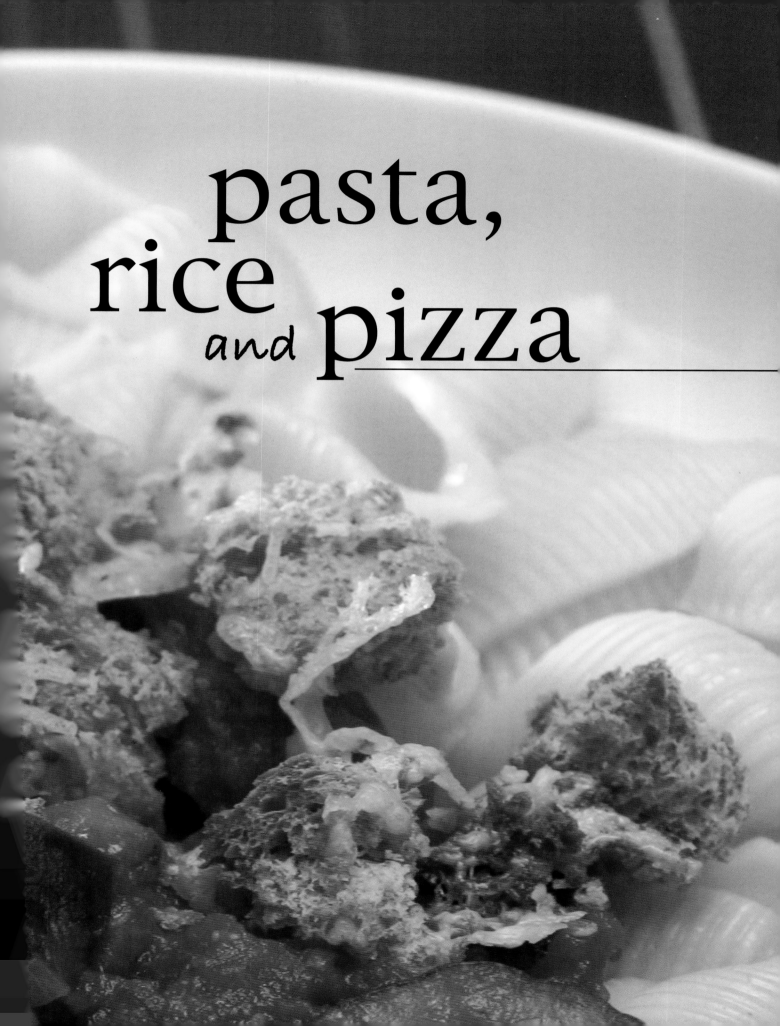

# pasta, rice and pizza

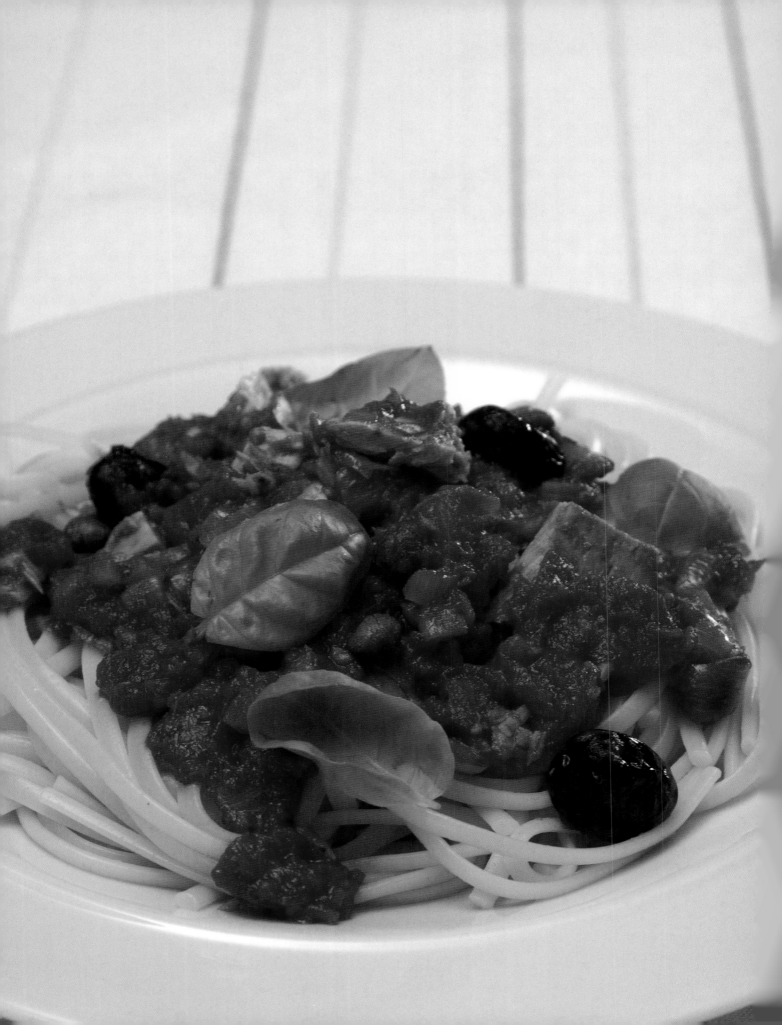

# Tuna Puttanesca

*Hot and spicy*

The combination of tuna and tomatoes makes this dish useful in providing vitamins C, D, E and B12.

## Serves 2

2 tsp olive oil
1 small onion, peeled and finely chopped
1 clove garlic, peeled and crushed
½ red chilli, sliced
½ tsp dried oregano
1 x 400g/14oz can tomatoes, chopped
1 x 200g/7oz can of tuna in spring water
200g/7oz spaghetti
8 black olives
1 tbsp capers
basil leaves to garnish

## Serves 4

4 tsp olive oil
1 onion, peeled and finely chopped
2 cloves garlic, peeled and crushed
1 red chilli, sliced
1 tsp dried oregano
2 x 400g/14oz cans tomatoes, chopped
2 x 200g/7oz cans of tuna in spring water
400g/14oz spaghetti
16 black olives
2 tbsp capers
basil leaves to garnish

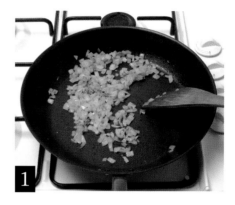

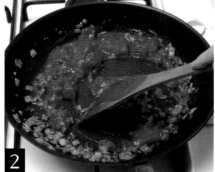

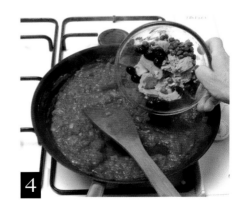

1 Fill a large saucepan with cold water and bring to the boil. Heat the oil in a frying pan and cook the onion over a moderate heat until softened. Add the garlic, chilli and oregano and cook, stirring, for 1–2 minutes. Do not let the garlic brown.

2 Add the tomatoes and stir well to mix. Bring gently to the boil, then reduce the heat to a gentle simmer.

3 Pour the pasta into the saucepan of boiling water

and return to the boil. When it is boiling, reduce the heat to a simmer and cook for 8 minutes, or according to the packet instructions.

4 Meanwhile, drain the tuna thoroughly and add to the tomato mixture with the olives and capers and stir to mix. Cook for a further 5 minutes.

5 Drain the pasta and divide between the serving plates. Spoon over the tuna and tomato sauce. Garnish with basil leaves to serve.

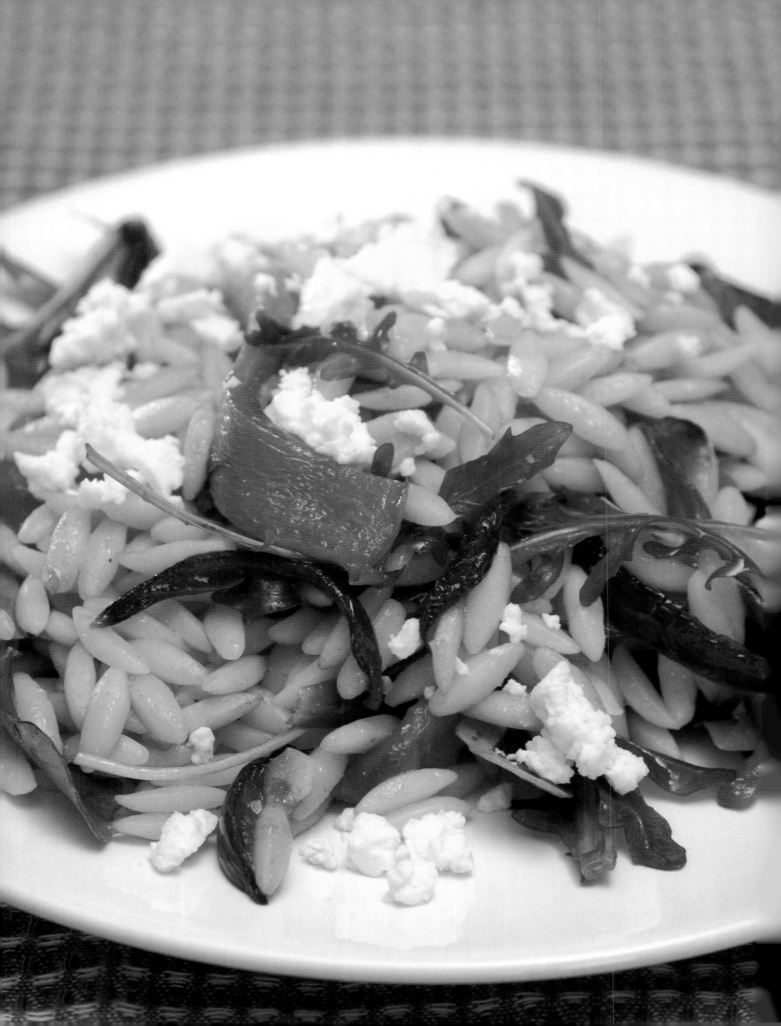

# Roast Pepper & Rocket Pasta

*vegetarian*

A colourful pasta dish that is a good source of vitamin C and carbohydrate.

## Serves 2

**1 large sweet pepper**
**2 tsp olive oil**
**1 small red onion, peeled and cut into thin wedges**
**1 clove garlic, peeled and finely chopped**
**200g/7oz orzo pasta**
**25g/1oz wild rocket**
**1 tbsp balsamic vinegar**
**40g/1½oz feta cheese**

## Serves 4

**2 large sweet peppers**
**4 tsp olive oil**
**1 large red onion, peeled and cut into thin wedges**
**2 cloves garlic, peeled and finely chopped**
**400g/14oz orzo pasta**
**50g/2oz wild rocket**
**2 tbsp balsamic vinegar**
**75g/3oz feta cheese**

1 Preheat the grill to high. Halve and deseed the pepper and slice into quarters. Cook under the preheated grill until the skins become charred. You may need to turn them to achieve this. Once they are cooked, remove them from the heat, place in a bowl and cover with cling film. Set to one side for 20 minutes.

2 Remove the cling film and peel the peppers, discarding the skins. Cut the flesh into thin strips and reserve.

3 Heat the oil in a frying pan and cook the onion over a moderate heat until it starts to turn golden in places. Add the garlic and the pepper strips and continue to cook over a gentle heat for 5 minutes, stirring from time to time.

4 Meanwhile fill a large saucepan with cold water and bring to the boil. Add the pasta and bring back to the boil. Now reduce the heat a little, cover, and cook for 8 minutes or according to the packet instructions

5 Drain the pasta and return to the saucepan. Add the onion and peppers, along with the rocket and balsamic vinegar. Toss to mix. Divide equally between the serving plates and crumble over the feta cheese to serve.

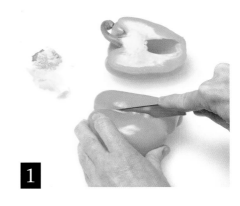

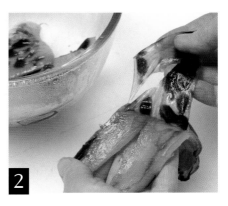

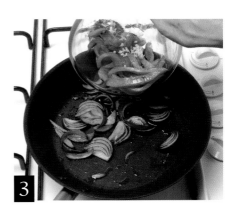

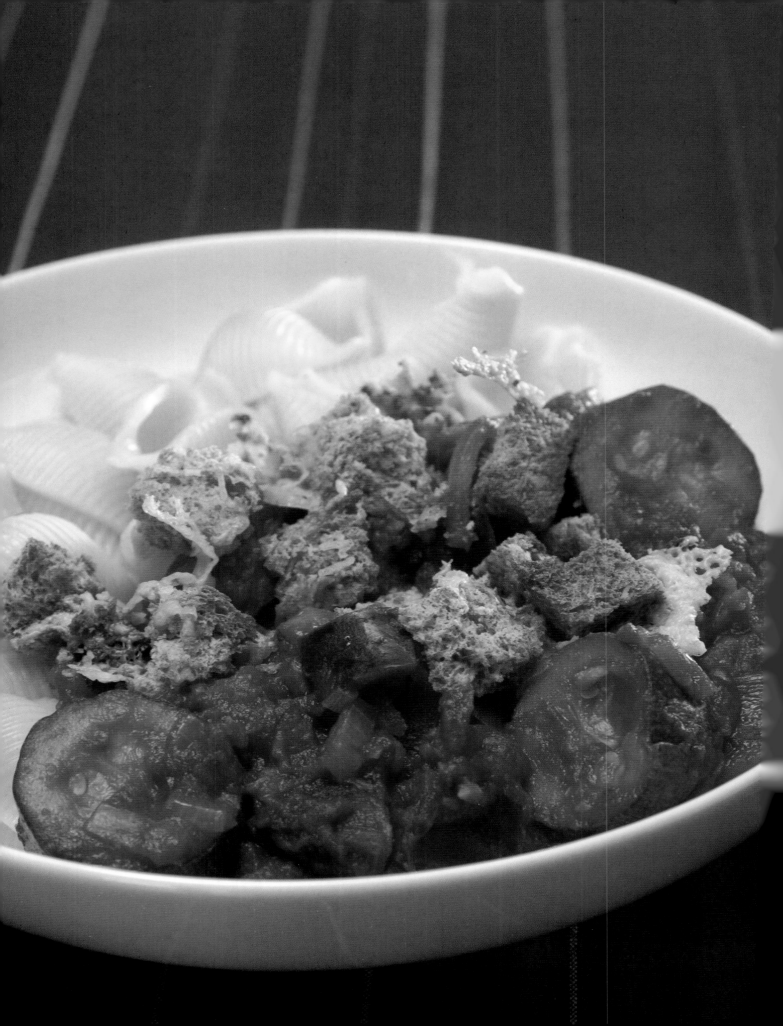

# Chilli Ratatouille with Pasta

*Hot and spicy*

This spiced vegetable stew is also good served with jacket potatoes. If you make too much, just store it in the fridge for up to 2 days and reheat until piping hot.

## Serves 2

- 1 tbsp olive oil
- 1 onion, peeled and sliced
- ½ green pepper, deseeded and cut into chunks
- 2 cloves garlic, peeled and finely chopped
- ¼ tsp crushed chilli flakes
- 1 courgette, trimmed and cut into chunks
- 1 small aubergine, trimmed and cut into chunks
- 1 x 400g/14oz can tomatoes, chopped
- 1 large thick slice brown bread
- 1 tbsp Parmesan cheese, finely grated
- 15g/½oz mature Cheddar cheese
- 200g/7oz pasta shells

## Serves 4

- 2 tbsp olive oil
- 1 large onion, peeled and sliced
- 1 green pepper, deseeded and cut into chunks
- 4 cloves garlic, peeled and finely chopped
- ½ tsp crushed chilli flakes
- 2 courgettes, trimmed and cut into chunks
- 1 aubergine, trimmed and cut into chunks
- 2 x 400g/14oz cans tomatoes, chopped
- 2 large thick slices brown bread
- 2 tbsp Parmesan cheese, finely grated
- 25g/1oz mature Cheddar cheese
- 400g/14oz pasta shells

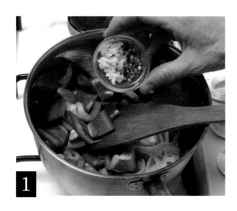

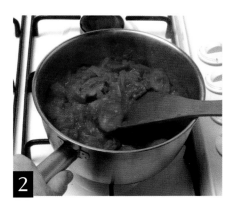

1 Preheat the oven to 190°C/375°F/Gas Mark 5. Heat the oil in a large saucepan and cook the onion over a moderate heat until it becomes transparent. Add the pepper, garlic and chilli flakes. Cook, stirring, for 2–3 minutes. Stir in the courgette and aubergine and cook for 4–5 minutes until they soften a little.

2 Add the tomatoes and bring gently to the boil. Reduce the heat to a gentle simmer and cook, covered, for about 30 minutes until reduced and thickened.

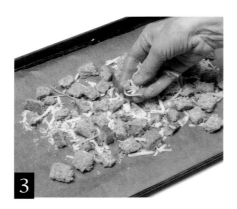

3

3 Meanwhile chop the bread into small chunks and spread over a baking sheet that has been lined with baking parchment or is non-stick. Sprinkle the cheeses over the bread. Bake in the preheated oven for 8–10 minutes until golden and crisp. Remove from the heat and allow to cool.

4 Bring a large saucepan of water to the boil and add the pasta. Cook according to the packet instructions and drain. Divide the pasta and sauce between the serving dishes and top with the crisp cheese crumbs. Serve.

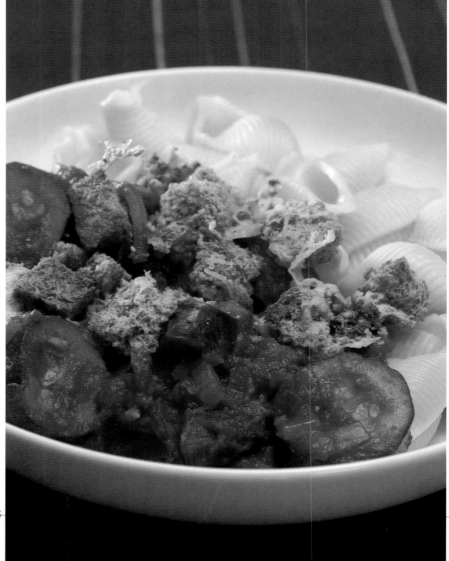

# Roasted Vegetables with Farfalle

*vegetarian*

In our house this is one of the most popular ways of cooking vegetables.

## Serves 2

300g/10½oz carrots, peeled and cut into thin batons
1 tbsp olive oil
1 red onion, peeled and cut into wedges
1 orange pepper, deseeded and cut into thin strips
150g/5oz courgettes, trimmed and cut into discs
3 cloves garlic, unpeeled
8 cherry tomatoes
2 tbsp balsamic vinegar
150g/5oz farfalle pasta
15g/½oz Parmesan, shaved into thin slices
freshly ground black pepper

## Serves 4

600g/1lb 5oz carrots, peeled and cut into thin batons
2 tbsp olive oil
2 red onions, peeled and cut into wedges
2 orange peppers, deseeded and cut into thin strips
275g/10oz courgettes, trimmed and cut into discs
6 cloves garlic, unpeeled
16 cherry tomatoes
4 tbsp balsamic vinegar
275g/10oz farfalle pasta
25g/1oz Parmesan, shaved into thin slices
freshly ground black pepper

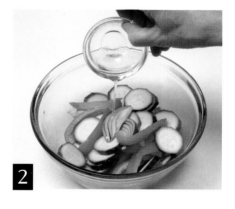

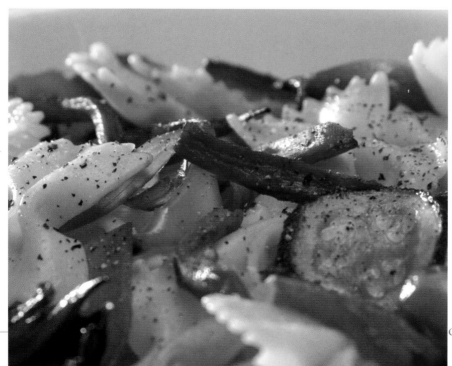

1 Preheat the oven to 200°F/400°C/Gas Mark 6. Place the carrots in a large mixing bowl and drizzle over half the oil, tossing well to coat. Tip the carrots into a large heavy-gauge roasting tin and spread out. Cook in the preheated oven for 15 minutes.

2 Add the red onion, pepper and courgette to the mixing bowl that held the carrots and drizzle over the remaining oil. Toss well to mix.

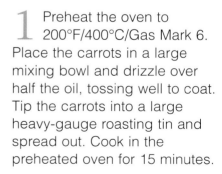

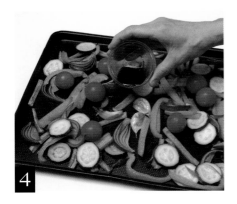

4

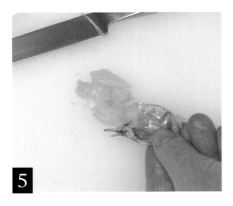

5

3 Add these to the roasting tin with the unpeeled garlic and toss well to mix. Return the tin to the oven and cook for 15 minutes.

4 Add the tomatoes and balsamic vinegar to the roasting tin and cook for a further 10 minutes.

5 Remove the tin from the oven and squeeze the softened flesh from the garlics' papery skin. Roughly chop the

flesh – it should be quite mushy – and add to the roasted vegetables.

6 Meanwhile bring a large pan of water to the boil and cook the pasta according to the packet instructions.

7 Toss the vegetables through the drained pasta. Serve topped with the Parmesan shavings and seasoned with black pepper.

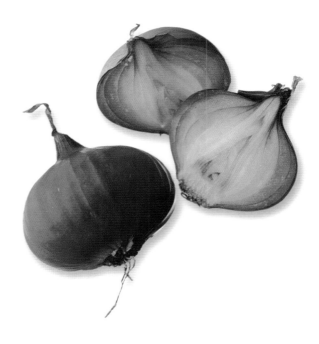

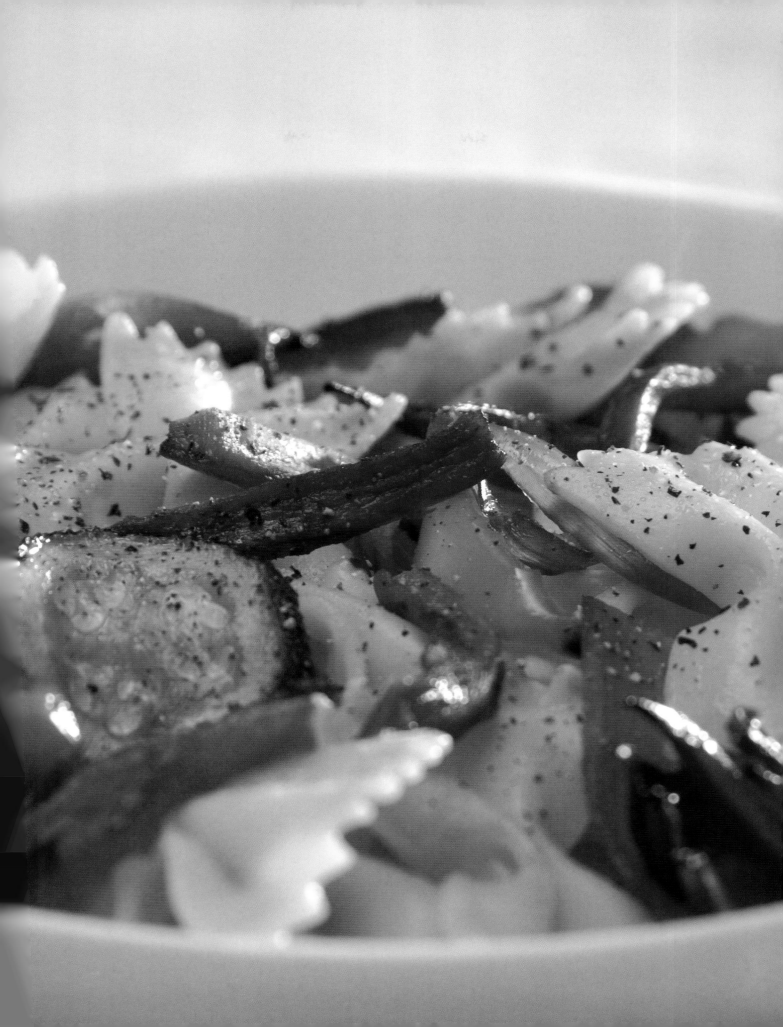

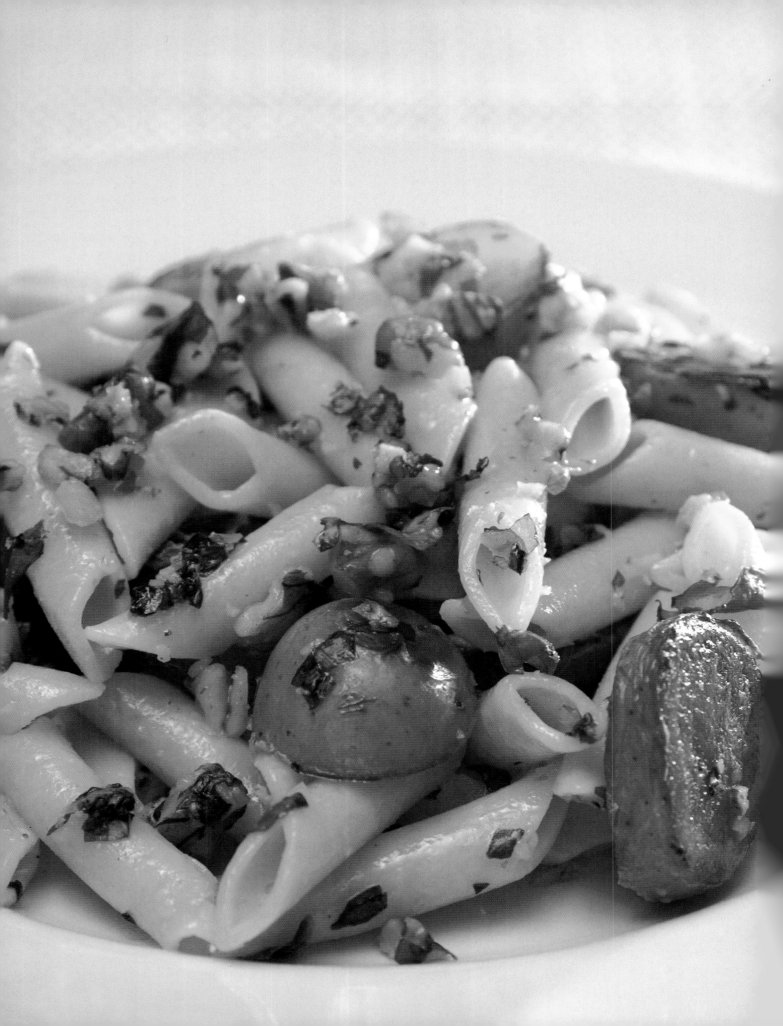

# Walnut & Potato Pasta

*vegetarian*

This is a useful meal to serve the sporting members of the family, as the high carbohydrate content is essential muscle fuel.

### Serves 2
**250g/9oz new potatoes**
**40g/1½oz walnuts**
**3 tbsp fresh basil**
**1 clove garlic, peeled**
**pinch of salt**
**25g/1oz Parmesan, finely grated**
**2 tbsp olive oil**
**150g/5oz penne pasta**

### Serves 4
**500g/1lb 2oz new potatoes**
**75g/3oz walnuts**
**6 tbsp fresh basil**
**2 cloves garlic, peeled**
**¼ tsp salt**
**50g/2oz Parmesan, finely grated**
**4 tbsp olive oil**
**275g/10oz penne pasta**

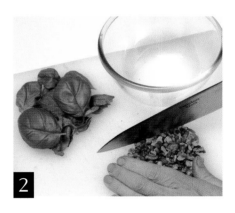

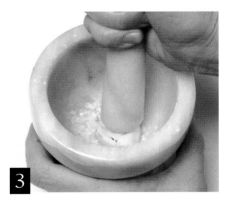

1 Bring a saucepan of water to the boil and cook the potatoes until just tender when tested with the tip of a knife. Remove from the heat and drain. When cool enough to handle, cut into thick slices.

2 Chop the walnuts and basil finely and place in a small mixing bowl.

3 Using a pestle and mortar, crush the garlic clove with the salt to a paste.

4 Add the paste to the walnuts and basil, along with the Parmesan and half the olive oil. Mix thoroughly and set to one side to allow the flavours to develop.

5 Heat the remaining olive oil in a frying pan large enough to take the potato slices in a single layer. Add the potatoes and cook over a moderate heat, turning from time to time until they become golden and crisp in places.

6 Meanwhile bring a large pan of water to the boil and cook the pasta according to the packet instructions.

7 Drain the pasta and return it to the saucepan. Add the crisped potatoes and the walnut and basil mixture. Toss well to mix. Serve.

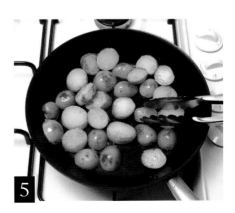

# Creamy Tomato & Thyme Shells

*vegetarian*

Ricotta is a relatively low-fat cheese and is a good source of calcium and protein.

### Serves 2

**2 tsp olive oil**
**1 small onion, peeled and finely chopped**
**2 cloves garlic, peeled and finely chopped**
**1 x 400g/14oz can tomatoes, chopped**
**a sprig of fresh thyme, plus a few leaves for garnish**
**200g/7oz pasta shells**
**100g/4oz ricotta**
**black pepper**

### Serves 4

**4 tsp olive oil**
**1 large onion, peeled and finely chopped**
**4 cloves garlic, peeled and finely chopped**
**2 x 400g/14oz cans tomatoes, chopped**
**a large sprig of fresh thyme, plus a few leaves for garnish**
**400g/14oz pasta shells**
**200g/7oz ricotta**
**black pepper**

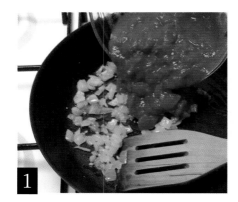

1 Heat the oil in a frying pan over a moderate heat and cook the onion until soft. Add the garlic and cook for 2 minutes, stirring. Pour in the tomatoes and bring gently to the boil.

2 Add the thyme and reduce the heat to a gentle simmer. Cook for about 15 minutes until the mixture thickens.

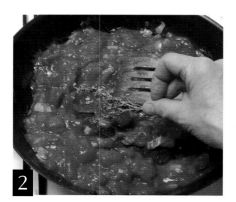

3 Bring a large pan of water to the boil and cook the pasta according to the packet instructions. Drain.

4 Add the ricotta to the thickened tomato and cook for a further 5 minutes. Divide the pasta between the serving plates and spoon over the sauce. Season with black pepper and garnish with fresh thyme leaves. Serve.

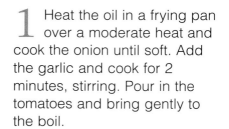

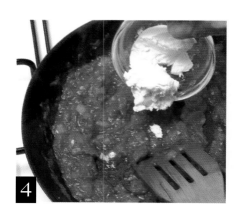

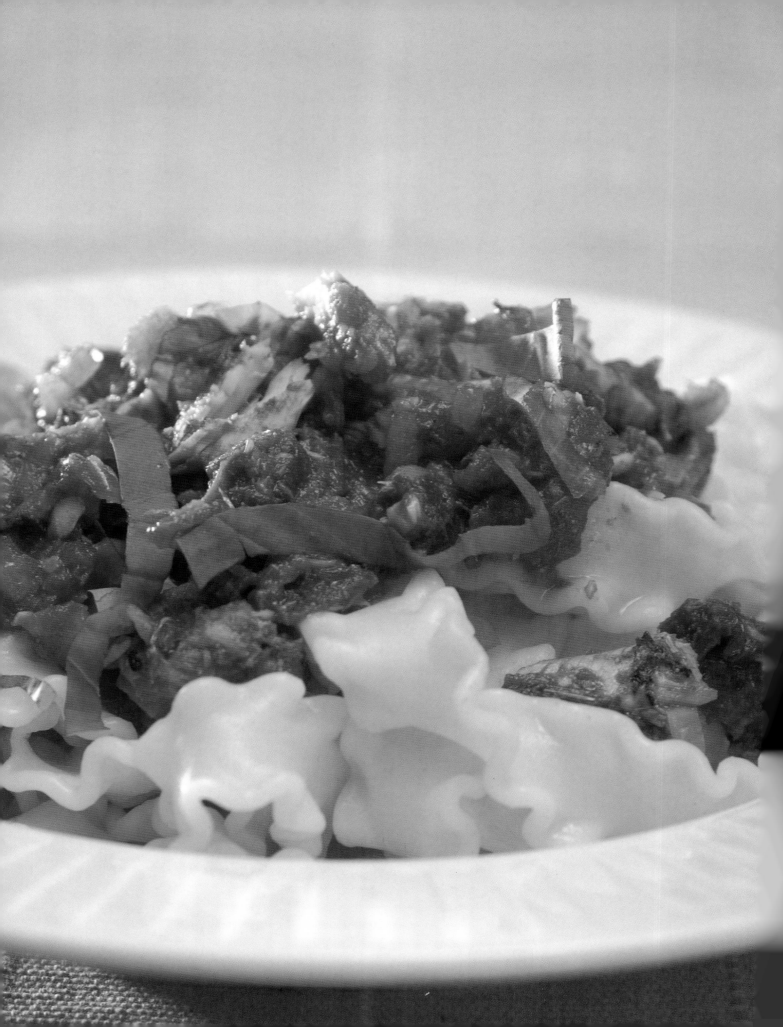

# Wilted Spinach & Prawn Pasta

*Easy Entertaining*

Prawns supply us with vitamin B12 and trace minerals, as well as being high in protein.

## Serves 2

**200g/7oz tagliatelle**
**1 tbsp olive oil**
**4 shallots, peeled and sliced**
**1 clove garlic, peeled and finely chopped**
**½ lemon**
**200g/7oz large raw peeled prawns**
**75g/3oz baby spinach leaves**
**freshly ground black pepper**

## Serves 4

**400g/14oz tagliatelle**
**2 tbsp olive oil**
**8 shallots, peeled and sliced**
**2 cloves garlic, peeled and finely chopped**
**1 lemon**
**400g/14oz large raw peeled prawns**
**150g/5oz baby spinach leaves**
**freshly ground black pepper**

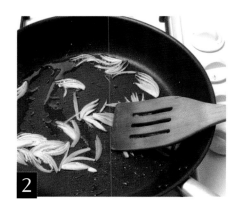

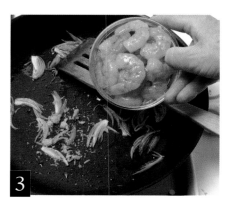

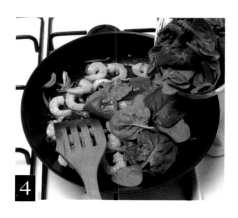

1 Bring a large saucepan of water to the boil and cook the pasta according to the packet instructions. Drain.

2 Meanwhile heat the oil in a frying pan and cook the sliced shallots over a moderate heat until they soften. Add the garlic and cook for a further 2 minutes.

3 Finely grate the zest from the lemon, squeeze the juice and add to the frying pan with the prawns. Cook, stirring from time to time, until the prawns are evenly pink.

4 Stir in the spinach and cook over a high heat until the spinach wilts. Remove from the heat and stir through the drained pasta. Season with freshly ground black pepper.

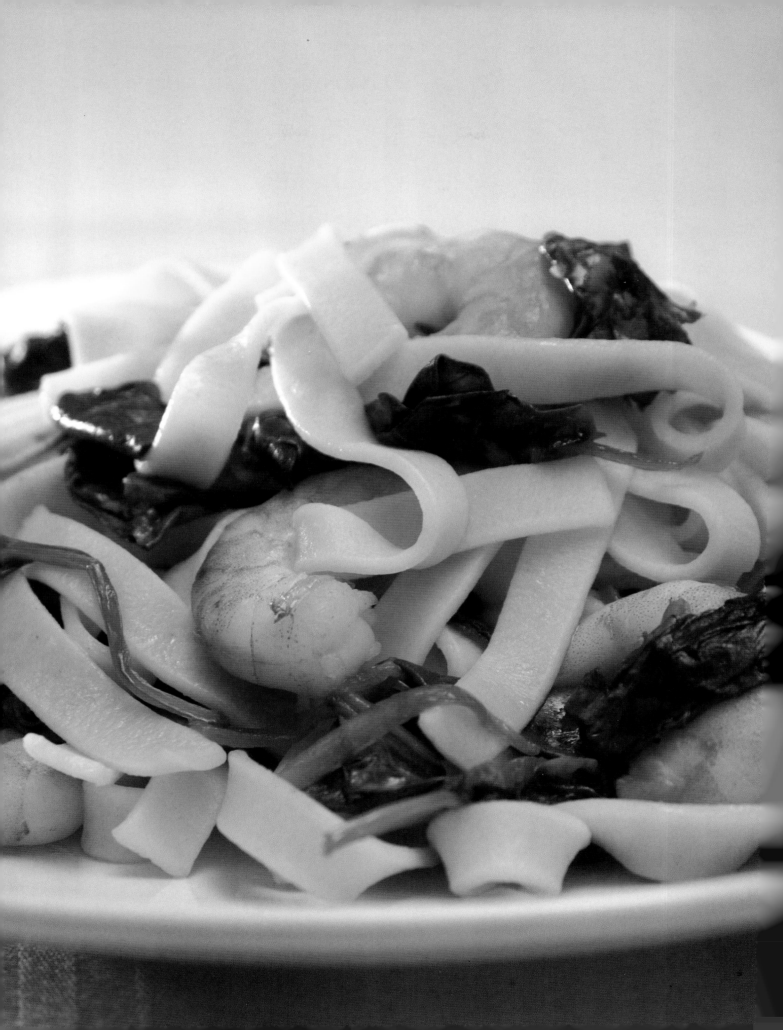

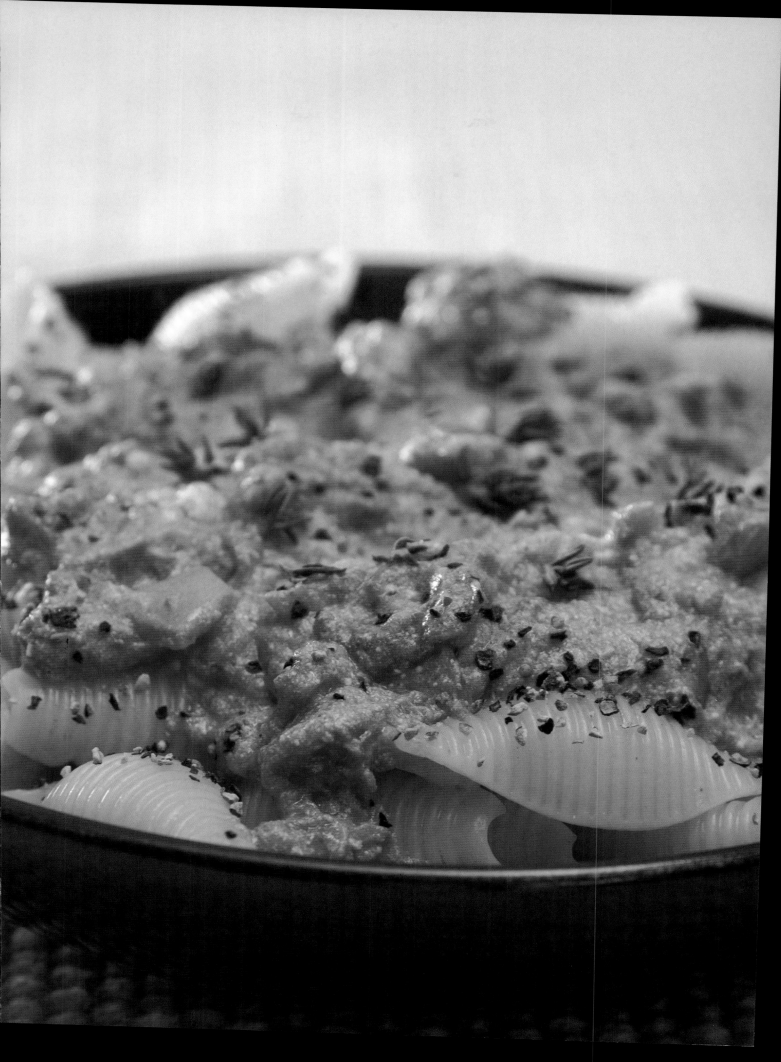

# Tomato & Sardine Pasta

*Quick and Easy*

Sardines provide us with omega-3 fatty acids.

## Serves 2

**1 tbsp olive oil**
**1 onion, peeled and finely chopped**
**2 cloves garlic, peeled and finely chopped**
**4 sun-dried tomatoes**
**1 x 200g/7oz can tomatoes, chopped**
**200g/7oz mafalde pasta**
**1 tsp red wine vinegar**
**1 x 125g/4½oz can sardines**
**3 tbsp fresh basil**

## Serves 4

**2 tbsp olive oil**
**1 large onion, peeled and finely chopped**
**4 cloves garlic, peeled and finely chopped**
**8 sun-dried tomatoes**
**1 x 400g/14oz can tomatoes, chopped**
**400g/14oz mafalde pasta**
**2 tsp red wine vinegar**
**2 x 125g/4½oz cans sardines**
**6 tbsp fresh basil**

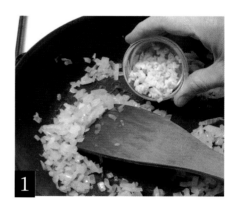

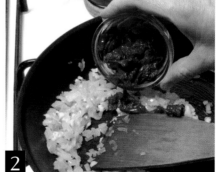

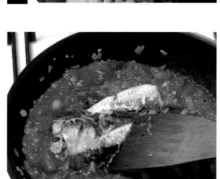

1 Heat the oil in a frying pan over a moderate heat and cook the onion until softened. Add the garlic and cook for 2–3 minutes until softened but not browned.

2 Roughly chop the sun-dried tomatoes and add to the pan, stirring well to mix.

3 Stir in the chopped tomatoes and cook at a gentle simmer until thickened.

4 Meanwhile bring a large saucepan of water to the boil and cook the pasta according to the packet instructions. Drain.

5 Add the vinegar and sardines to the frying pan and cook, stirring, for 2–3 minutes until piping hot. Serve spooned over the pasta and sprinkled with the shredded basil.

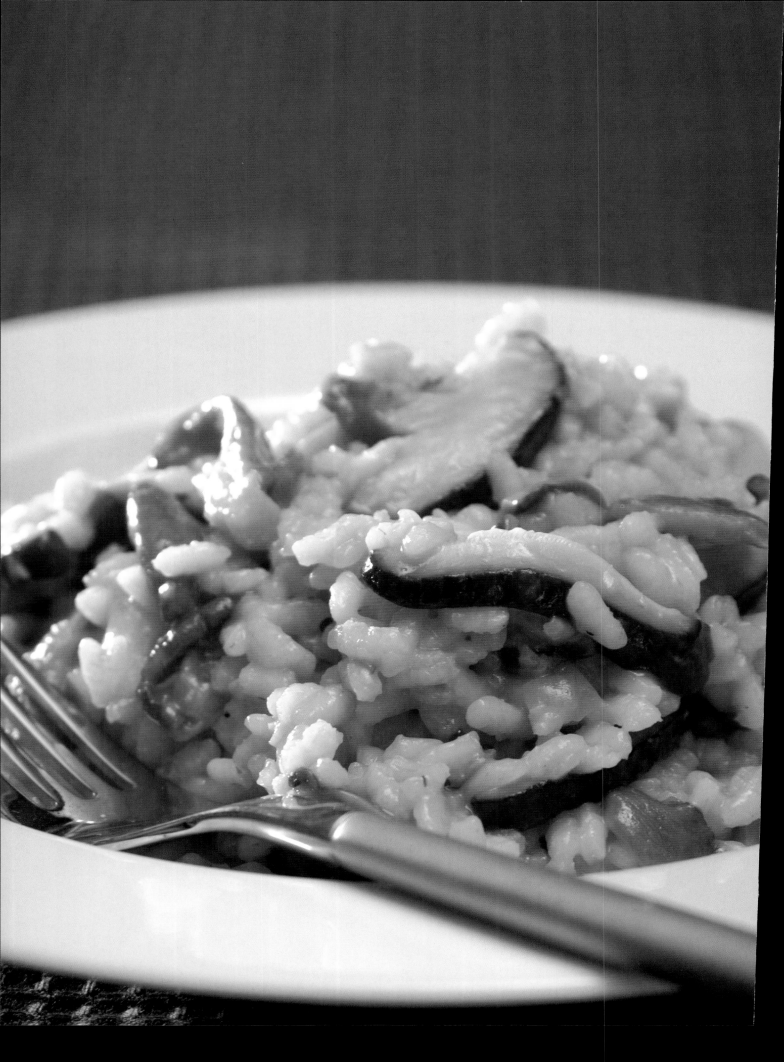

# Mushroom Risotto

*One Pot*

A simple, satisfying supper dish. Just serve with a light salad or vegetable of your choice.

## Serves 2

**2 tsp olive oil**
**15g/½oz butter**
**2 shallots, peeled and finely chopped**
**1 small clove garlic, peeled and finely chopped**
**500ml/18fl oz vegetable stock**
**225g/8oz mixed mushrooms, sliced if large**
**150g/5oz Arborio rice**
**15g/½oz Parmesan, finely grated**
**salt and freshly ground black pepper to taste**

## Serves 4

**4 tsp olive oil**
**25g/1oz butter**
**4 shallots, peeled and finely chopped**
**1 clove garlic, peeled and finely chopped**
**1l/1¾pt vegetable stock**
**450g/1lb mixed mushrooms, sliced if large**
**300g/10½oz Arborio rice**
**25g/1oz Parmesan, finely grated**
**salt and freshly ground black pepper to taste**

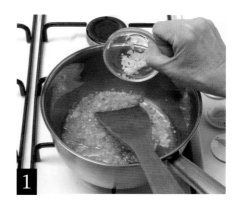

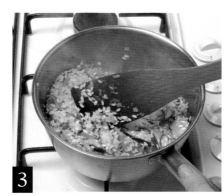

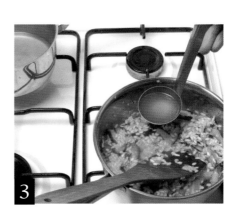

1 Heat the oil and the butter in a large saucepan. Add the shallots and cook over a moderate heat until they become transparent and softened. Add the garlic and cook for a further minute.

2 Place the stock in a saucepan, bring to the boil, and reduce the heat to a very gentle simmer. Cover.

3 Stir the mushrooms into the shallots and cook for 4–5 minutes. Add the rice and stir well to coat. Cook for 1–2 minutes. Add three to four ladles of the hot stock, stirring well to mix. Cook, stirring gently, until the liquid has almost been absorbed before adding another three to four ladles of the hot stock.

4 Continue cooking in this way until the mixture is thick and creamy and the rice is tender but not soft – risotto should have a little "bite" to it. You may not need all the hot stock, just keep adding it until the risotto is to your liking.

5 Remove from the heat and add the Parmesan, stirring quickly to mix. Season with salt and freshly ground black pepper to taste and serve.

# Beetroot Risotto

*One Pot*

Parmesan is a high-fat cheese but it is so rich in flavour that a little goes a long way. It is a good source of calcium, which is essential in a healthy diet.

## Serves 2

**225g/8oz ready-cooked beetroot**
**2 tsp olive oil**
**15g/½oz butter**
**1 red onion, peeled and finely chopped**
**500ml/18fl oz vegetable stock**
**150g/5oz brown rice**
**15g/½oz Parmesan shavings**
**salt and freshly ground black pepper to taste**

## Serves 4

**450g/1lb ready-cooked beetroot**
**4 tsp olive oil**
**25g/1oz butter**
**1 large red onion, peeled and finely chopped**
**1l/1¾pt vegetable stock**
**300g/10½oz brown rice**
**25g/1oz Parmesan shavings**
**salt and freshly ground black pepper to taste**

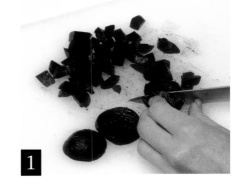

1 Cut the beetroot into small dice and set to one side. Heat the oil and butter in a large saucepan over a moderate heat. Add the red onion and cook over a moderate heat until it is transparent and softened. Place the stock in a saucepan, bring to the boil, then reduce the heat to a very gentle simmer. Cover.

2 Add the rice and stir well to coat in the mixture. Cook for 1–2 minutes. Add three to four ladles of the hot stock to the rice mixture, stirring well to mix. Cook, stirring gently, until the liquid has almost been absorbed before adding another three to four ladles of the hot stock.

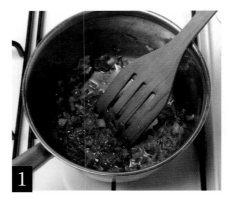

3 When almost half the stock has been added, stir in the beetroot. Continue adding the stock until the rice is tender and most of the liquid has been absorbed. You may not need all the hot stock, just keep adding it until the risotto is to your liking. Sprinkle with the Parmesan, season and serve.

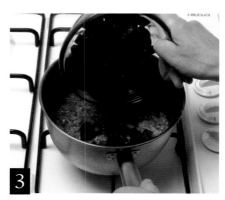

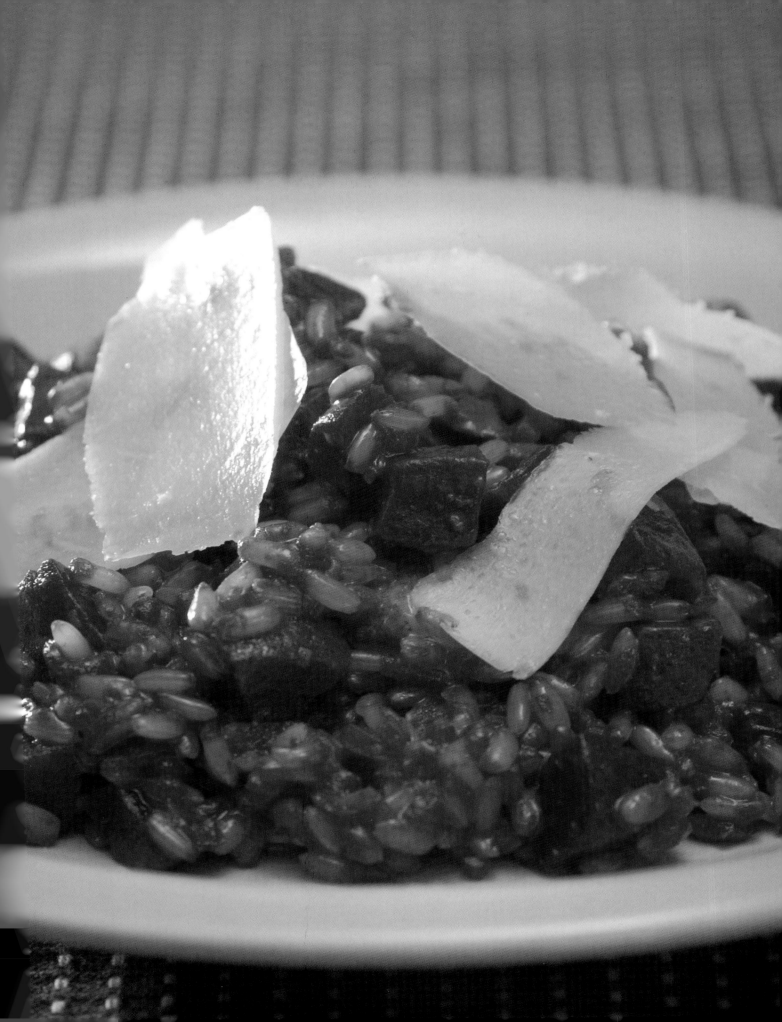

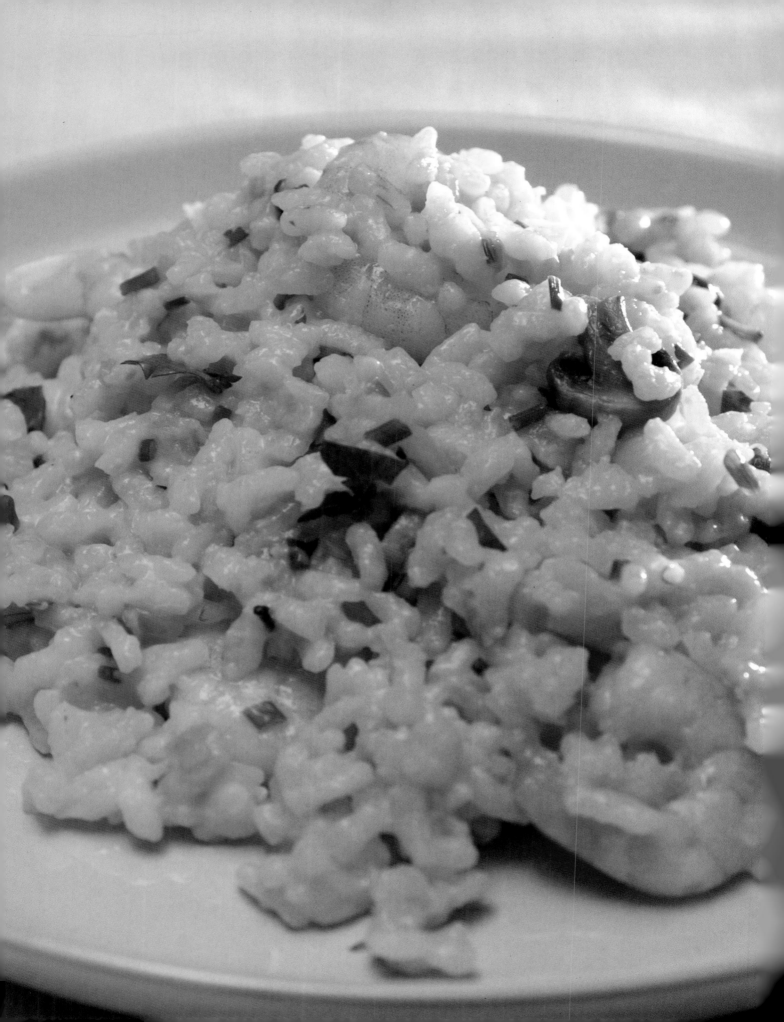

# Prawn Risotto

*Easy Entertaining*

Rice is eaten worldwide and for good reason, since it is gluten free, contains no cholesterol and is an excellent form of carbohydrate.

## Serves 2

**150g/5oz whole prawns**
**1 tbsp olive oil**
**1 onion, peeled and chopped**
**1 small clove garlic, peeled and crushed**
**50g/2oz button mushrooms, thinly sliced**
**150g/5oz Arborio rice**
**1 tbsp fresh chives, chopped**
**1 tbsp fresh parsley, chopped**
**¼ tsp lemon zest**

## Serves 4

**275g/10oz whole prawns**
**2 tbsp olive oil**
**1 large onion, peeled and chopped**
**1 clove garlic, peeled and crushed**
**100g/4oz button mushrooms, thinly sliced**
**275g/10oz Arborio rice**
**2 tbsp fresh chives, chopped**
**2 tbsp fresh parsley, chopped**
**½ tsp lemon zest**

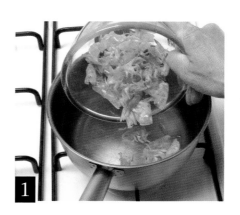

1 Peel the prawns, reserving the shells. Place them in a cool place while you prepare the stock. Pour 1l/1¾pt (2l/3¼pt) cold water into a large saucepan and add the prawn shells. Bring gently to the boil and cook at a rolling boil until the liquid has reduced by a third. Strain, discarding the shells. Return the stock to the pan and keep warm.

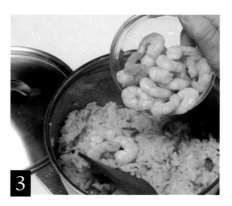

2 Heat the oil in a large saucepan and cook the onion and garlic until softened. Add the mushrooms and continue to cook for 3–4 minutes until softened.

3 Stir in the rice and cook for 1 minute, stirring well to coat in the oil and mushroom mixture. Start adding the warm stock, three to four ladles at a time, stirring as you do so. Cook until almost all the stock has been absorbed, then add more. Continue doing this until the rice is tender and creamy in consistency. Add the prawns with the final addition of stock and stir well to mix. You may not need all the stock. If, however, you need more, just add a little warm water.

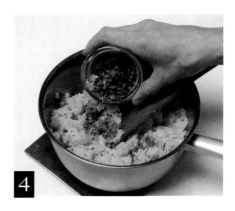

4 Remove the lid and stir through the chopped herbs and lemon zest. Serve.

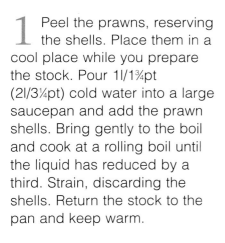

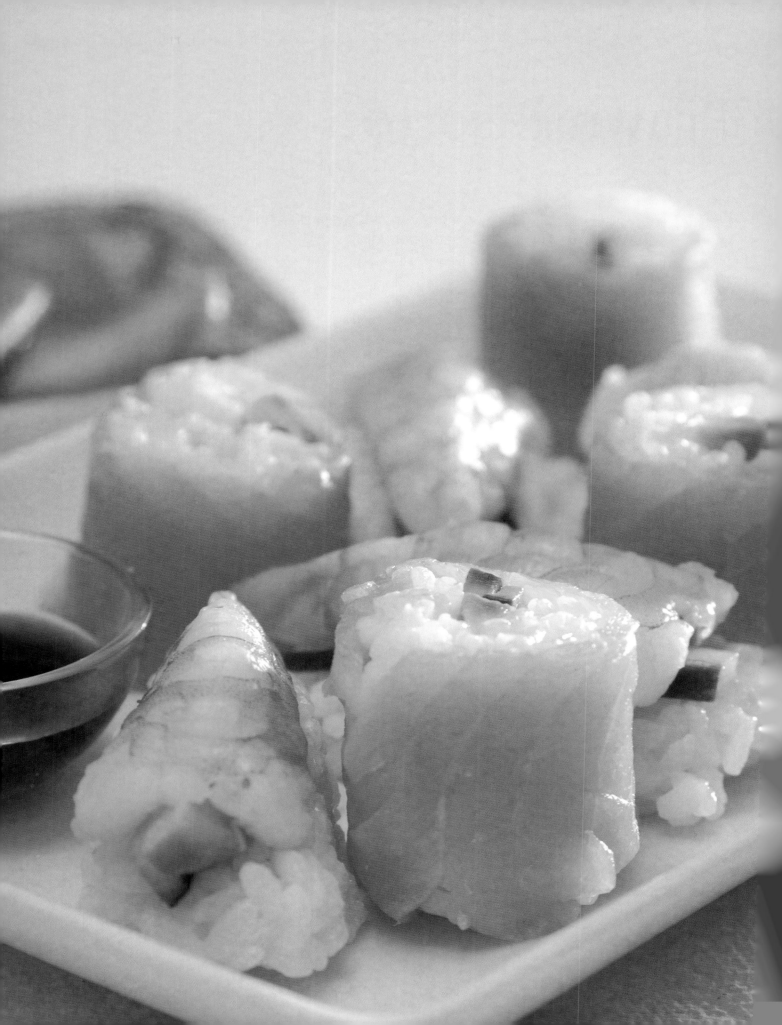

# Prawn & Smoked Salmon Sushi

## *Family Favourite*

These are a bit fiddly but fun. Try experimenting with your own shapes and vegetable combinations.

### Serves 2

**100g/4oz sushi rice**
**2 tbsp rice wine vinegar**
**2 tsp caster sugar**
**½ tsp salt**
**8 large peeled, cooked tiger prawns**
**100g/4oz smoked salmon**
**¼ cucumber**
**½ avocado**
**½ lemon, juiced**
**1 tsp wasabi**
**pickled ginger and soy sauce to serve**

### Serves 4

**225g/8oz sushi rice**
**4 tbsp rice wine vinegar**
**4 tsp caster sugar**
**1 tsp salt**
**16 large peeled, cooked tiger prawns**
**225g/8oz smoked salmon**
**½ cucumber**
**1 avocado**
**1 lemon, juiced**
**1 tsp wasabi**
**pickled ginger and soy sauce to serve**

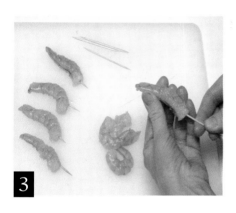

1 Place the rice in a sieve and wash thoroughly under cold running water until the water runs clear. Set the rice to one side to drain. Heat the vinegar, sugar and salt in a small pan over a very gentle heat, stirring until the sugar and salt have dissolved. Remove from the heat and leave to cool.

2 Place the drained rice in a saucepan with 100ml/3½fl oz (200ml/7fl oz) cold water. Bring to the boil, reduce the heat to a gentle simmer and cook, covered, for 15 minutes.

Remove from the heat but keep covered. Leave to stand for 10 minutes. Turn the rice out onto a large plate and sprinkle over the vinegar mixture. Toss the mixture gently to mix, then fan to cool.

3 Prepare the remaining ingredients ready to assemble the sushi. Push a cocktail stick through the length of the prawn to straighten it as much as possible. Cook the prawns in a little boiling water until they are pink and piping hot.

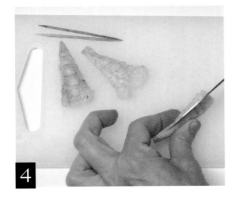

4 Remove from the heat and when cool enough to handle remove the cocktail sticks and butterfly the prawns, cutting along their inner edge to open them out flat.

5 Cut the smoked salmon into 10cm/4in x 5cm/2in strips and set to one side. Cut the cucumber in half, deseed and slice the flesh into fine strips. Peel the avocado and cut into thin batons, sprinkle with the lemon juice and set to one side.

6 To make the smoked salmon sushi, take 1 tbsp of the cooled rice and shape it into a roll that will fit along the short side of a piece of salmon. Smear a little wasabi down the rice and lay a piece of cucumber and avocado on this, pressing them lightly into the rice. Roll the salmon around the rice and cut the roll in half. Repeat with the remaining salmon until it is all used up.

7 To make the prawn sushi, take 1 tbsp of the rice and shape it roughly with your hands to the size of one of the prawns. Smear a little wasabi on the top edge. Place a piece of the cucumber and avocado on top and then shape the cut prawn around this to enclose. Repeat with the remaining prawns. Serve with the pickled ginger and soy sauce.

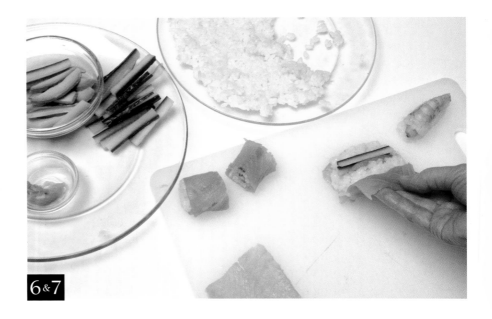

# Paella

One Pot

A colourful, tasty meal in one.

## Serves 2

175g/6oz live mussels
1 tbsp olive oil
2 chicken drumsticks, skin
    removed
1 onion, peeled and chopped
1 clove garlic, peeled and
    finely chopped
½ red pepper, deseeded
    and chopped
½ tbsp paprika
½ tsp turmeric
175g/6oz paella rice
500ml/18fl oz chicken stock
100g/4oz frozen peas
50g/2oz large peeled prawns
½ lemon cut into wedges

## Serves 4

350g/12oz live mussels
2 tbsp olive oil
4 chicken drumsticks, skin
    removed
1 large onion, peeled and
    chopped
2 cloves garlic, peeled and
    finely chopped
1 red pepper, deseeded and
    chopped
1 tbsp paprika
1 tsp turmeric
350g/12oz paella rice
1l/1¾pt chicken stock
200g/7oz frozen peas
100g/4oz large peeled prawns
1 lemon cut into wedges

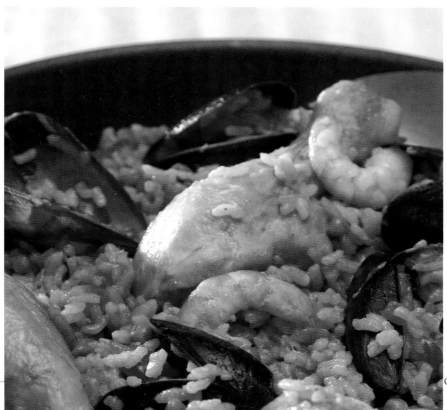

1 Wash the mussels thoroughly, removing any barnacles by scraping them. Pull away any "hairy beards" that may be protruding from them. Discard any mussels that do not shut when you tap their shells sharply.

2 Heat the oil in a large frying pan and cook the chicken drumsticks over a moderate heat, turning until evenly browned. Remove from the pan and keep warm.

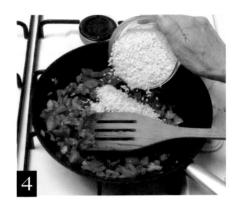

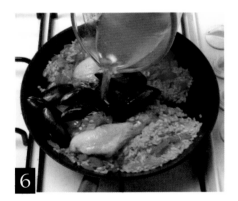

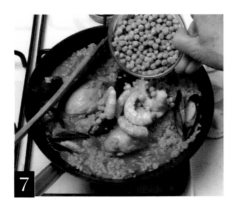

3 Add the onion and garlic to the pan and cook, stirring from time to time, until the onion is softened and starting to turn golden in places. Add the chopped red pepper and cook for a further 4–5 minutes.

4 Add the paprika and turmeric and cook for 1 minute, stirring. Add the rice and stir to coat in the spiced oil and onion mixture.

5 Return the chicken to the pan and pour in half of the chicken stock. Bring gently to the boil.

6 When the stock has almost all been absorbed, add the mussels to the pan along with the remaining stock. Bring to the boil and reduce the heat to a gentle simmer. Cook, covered, for about 8 minutes.

7 Remove the lid and stir in the peas and prawns. Simmer gently for 3–4 minutes. Discard any mussels that have not fully opened. Serve with lemon wedges for squeezing.

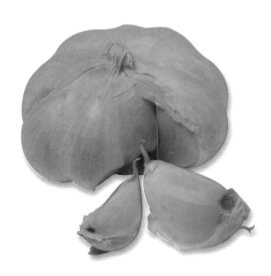

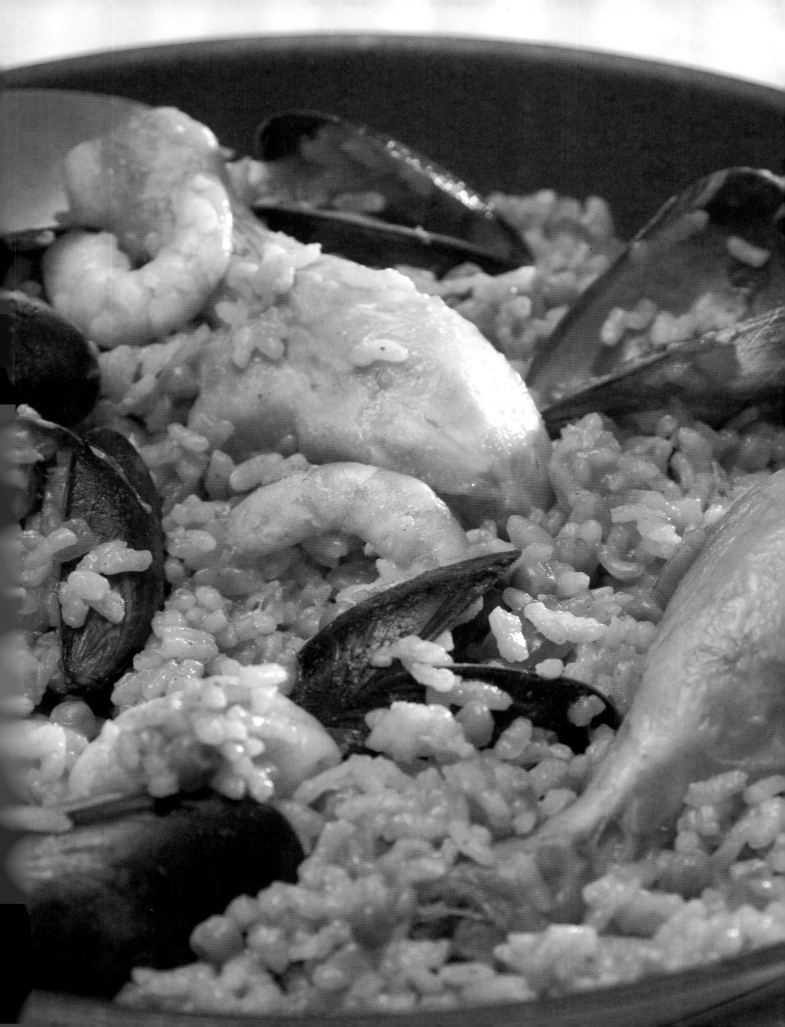

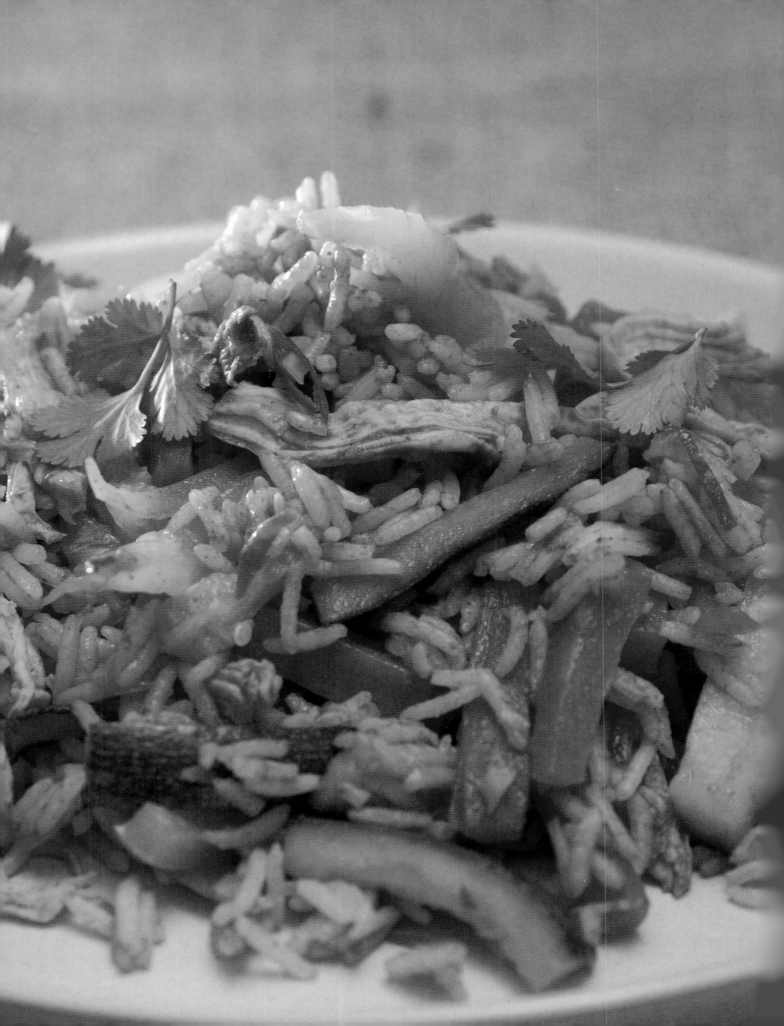

# Chicken Spiced Rice

*Hot and spicy*

This is just as tasty hot or cold. Handy to pack in lunch boxes

**Serves 2**

125g/4½oz basmati rice
2 tsp sunflower oil
1 small onion, peeled and
    sliced into thin wedges
1 clove garlic, peeled and
    finely chopped
½-1 fresh red chilli
    according to taste
1cm/½in ginger, peeled and
    finely grated
125g/4½oz carrots, peeled
    and coarsely grated
½ yellow pepper, deseeded
    and thinly sliced
1 medium courgette, trimmed
    and sliced into thin batons
½ tbsp paprika
1 large chicken breast,
    cooked and shredded
1½ tbsp tomato ketchup
½ tbsp dark soy sauce
fresh coriander to garnish
freshly ground black pepper
    to taste

**Serves 4**

250g/9oz basmati rice
4 tsp sunflower oil
1 onion, peeled and sliced
    into thin wedges
2 cloves garlic, peeled and
    finely chopped
1-2 fresh red chillies
    according to taste
2.5cm/1in ginger, peeled and
    finely grated
250g/9oz carrots, peeled and
    coarsely grated
1 yellow pepper, deseeded
    and thinly sliced
1 large courgette, trimmed
    and sliced into thin batons
1 tbsp paprika
2 large chicken breasts,
    cooked and shredded
3 tbsp tomato ketchup
1 tbsp dark soy sauce
fresh coriander to garnish
freshly ground black pepper
    to taste

1 Rinse the rice under cold running water and drain thoroughly. Now place the rice in a saucepan with 300ml/½pt (600ml/1pt) water and bring to the boil. Reduce the heat to a gentle simmer and cover with a well-fitting lid. Cook for 8–10 minutes or until all the liquid has been absorbed. Fork through to separate the rice and set to one side while you prepare the rest of the dish.

2 Heat the oil in a wok or large frying pan and cook the onion until it softens. Add the garlic, chilli and ginger and continue to cook, stirring, for 2–3 minutes.

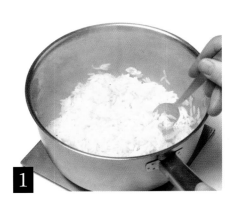

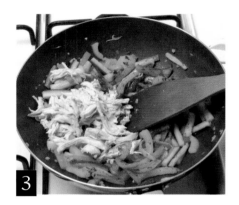

3 Stir in the carrots, pepper and courgette. Stir-fry for 3–4 minutes. Sprinkle over the paprika and cook for 1 minute. Add the cooked rice and mix thoroughly. Stir in the shredded chicken.

4 Mix the tomato ketchup and soy sauce with 1 (2) tbsp water and pour over the rice mixture, stirring as you do so. Continue to cook, stirring, for 5 minutes until the mixture is piping hot. Season to taste and serve garnished with coriander.

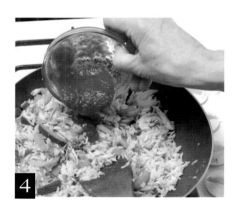

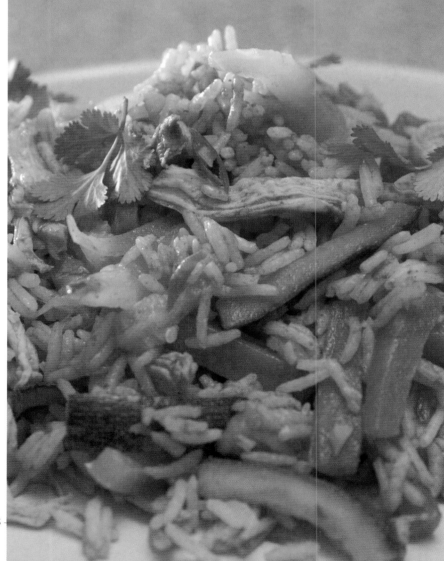

# Pizza

Pizza is always a hit. Making your own with wholemeal flour and a topping of fresh vegetables makes this one good for you too.

### Serves 2

**175g/6oz wholemeal flour**
**pinch sugar**
**¼ tsp salt**
**½ tsp dried easy-action**
    **yeast**
**1 tbsp olive oil**
**½ red pepper, deseeded**
    **and sliced**
**½ red onion, peeled and**
    **sliced into thin wedges**
**1 courgette, trimmed and**
    **sliced**
**50g/2oz cherry tomatoes**
**coarse cornmeal or**
    **polenta for sprinkling**
**salt and freshly ground black**
    **pepper to taste**
**50g/2oz mozzarella, grated**

### Serves 2-4

**350g/12oz wholemeal flour**
**¼ tsp sugar**
**½ tsp salt**
**1 tsp dried easy-action yeast**
**2 tbsp olive oil**
**1 red pepper, deseeded and**
    **sliced**
**1 red onion, peeled and**
    **sliced into thin wedges**
**1 large courgette, trimmed**
    **and sliced**
**100g/4oz cherry tomatoes**
**coarse cornmeal or**
    **polenta for sprinkling**
**salt and freshly ground black**
    **pepper to taste**
**100g/4oz mozzarella, grated**

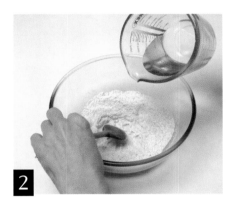

1 Place the flour in a mixing bowl and add the sugar and salt. Stir to mix. Sprinkle over the yeast and mix.

2 Stir half of the olive oil into 150ml/¼pt (300ml/½pt) tepid water. Make a hollow in the flour and pour in the water and oil mix, drawing the flour in from the sides to make a smooth dough. Turn out onto a lightly floured surface and knead for 10 minutes, until the dough is smooth and springy to the touch. Return to the mixing bowl and cover with cling film. Leave in a warm place for 1–2 hours or until the dough has doubled in size.

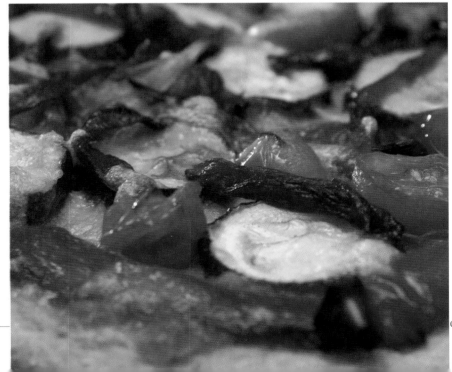

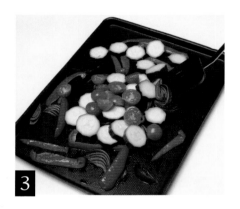

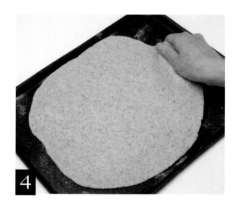

3 Preheat the oven to 200°C/400°F/Gas Mark 6. Place the red pepper and onion in a baking tray and drizzle with the remaining oil. Cook in the preheated oven for 15 minutes. Add the courgette and tomatoes and toss to mix in the oil that remains in the baking tray. Cook for a further 10 minutes. Remove and set to one side.

4 Increase the oven temperature to 240°C/475°F/Gas Mark 9. Knead the risen dough briefly, then roll out to form 1 (2) 35cm/14in rounds. Sprinkle a heavy-gauge baking sheet with a little cornmeal, then place the dough round on the prepared baking sheet. Top with the roasted vegetables and season. Sprinkle over the mozzarella cheese. Bake in the preheated oven for 15 minutes until golden and crisp. Serve cut into thick wedges.

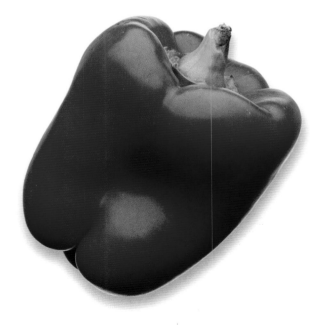

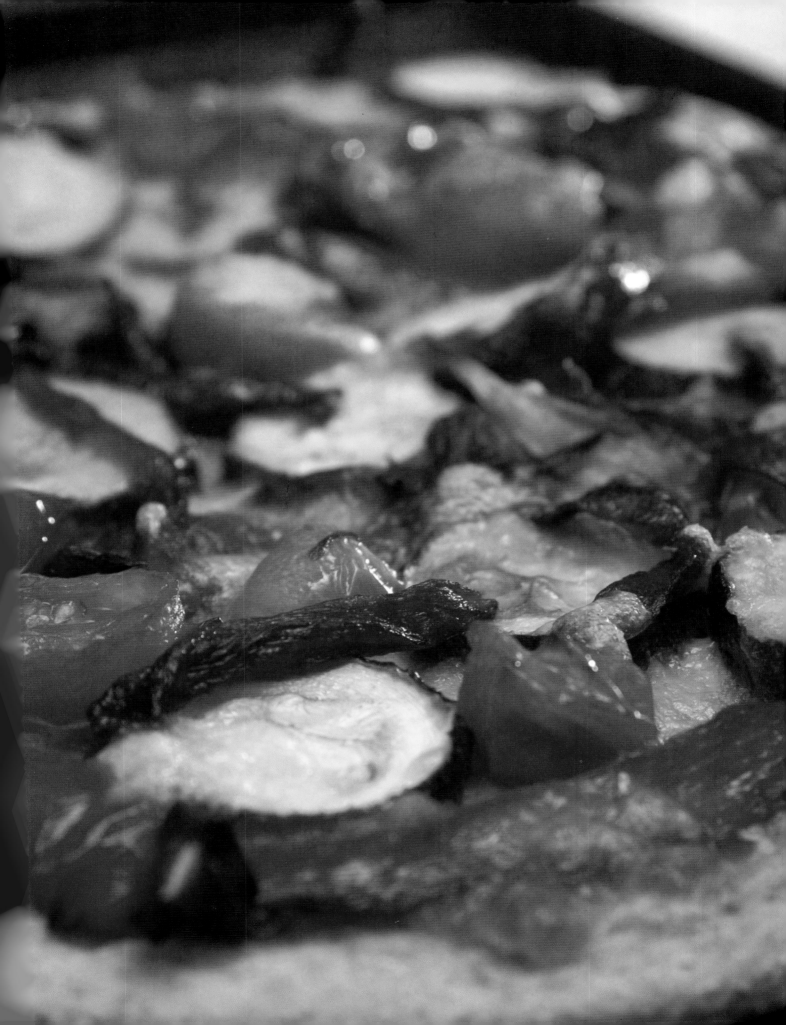

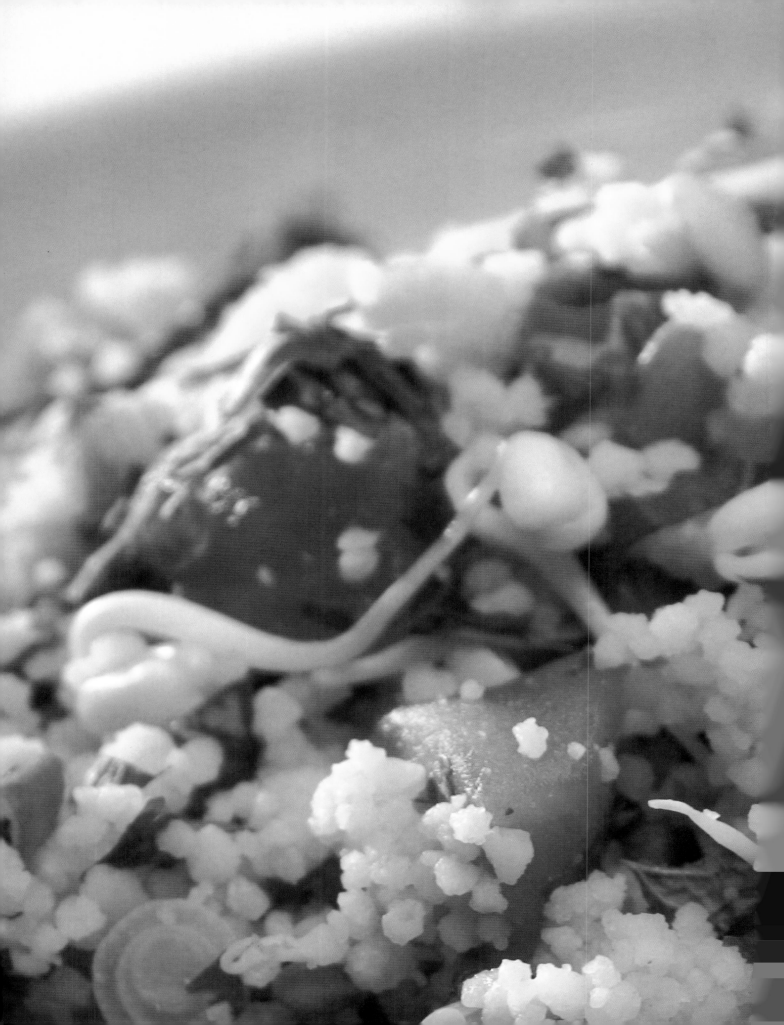

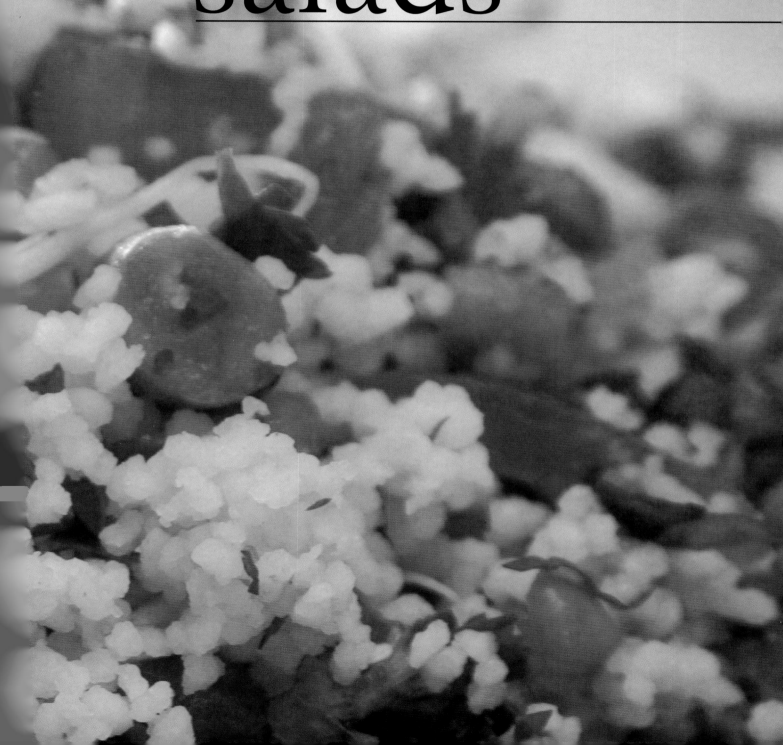

# vegetables
## salads _and_

# Layered Root Loaf

*Easy Entertaining*

This savoury loaf is a good source of vitamin C, E, folate and fibre.

### Serves 4-6

**Oil for spraying**
**400g/14oz potatoes, peeled**
**400g/14oz parsnips, peeled**
**400g/14oz sweet potato, peeled**
**1 egg**
**1 clove garlic, finely chopped**
**1 tbsp fresh chives, chopped**
**1 tbsp fresh parsley, chopped**
**150ml/¼pt vegetable stock**
**salt and freshly ground black pepper to taste**

1 Lightly oil and base-line a 23 x 12.5 x 7.5cm (9 x 5 x 3in) loaf tin. Preheat the oven to 190°C/ 375°F/ Gas Mark 5. Slice all the vegetables as thinly as possible. This is best done on a mandolin or in a food processor with a thin cutting disc. If using a sharp knife, try to get them all a similar thickness.

2 In a jug, beat the egg together with the garlic and chopped herbs. Add the vegetable stock and mix again. Place a single layer of the potatoes in the bottom of the prepared tin. Top these with a layer of the parsnips followed by a layer of the sweet potato. Continue in this way, repeating the layers and seasoning lightly every few layers, until all the vegetables have been used up.

3 Pour the egg and stock mixture evenly over the layered vegetables. It is best to do this slowly so the liquid has time to soak down through the layers.

4 Cover with foil, pinching around the edges to seal.

5 Bake in the preheated oven for 1½ hours. Remove the foil and return to the oven for a further 30–40 minutes. Test with a knife to check the loaf is tender and cooked through. Turn out onto a plate and serve cut in slices.

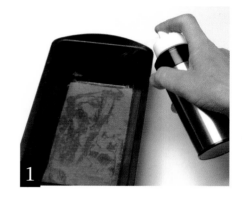

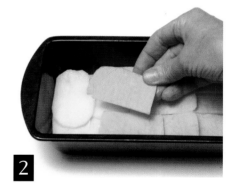

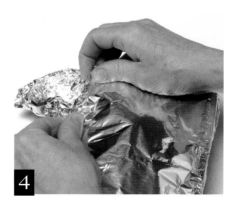

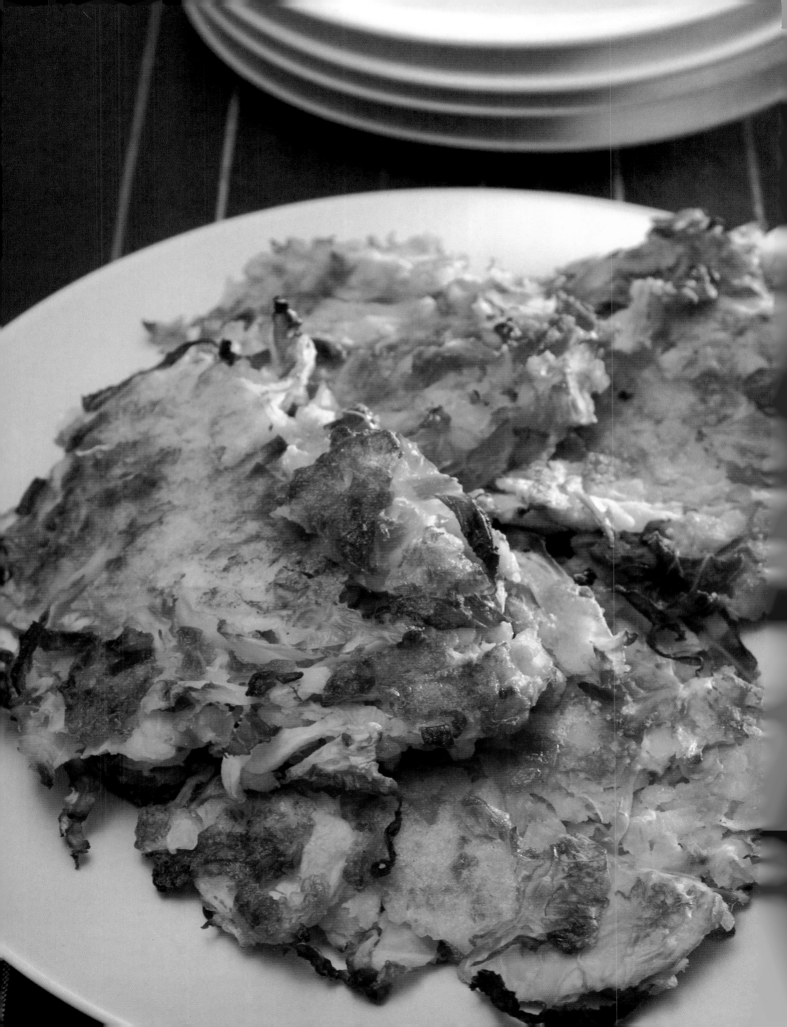

# Oven-baked Bubble & Squeak

*Children's Choice*

If you have any leftover cooked vegetables, this is a perfect way to make good use of them – just omit the cabbage and instead mix the vegetables into the mashed potato at the end of step 1.

## Serves 2

**400g/14oz potatoes, peeled and cut into chunks**
**300g/10½oz green cabbage, shredded**
**15g/½oz butter**
**2 tsp oil**
**1/2 small onion, peeled and very finely chopped**
**1 clove garlic, peeled and crushed**
**1½ tbsp Worcestershire sauce**

## Serves 4

**800g/1lb 12oz potatoes, peeled and cut into chunks**
**600g/1lb 5oz green cabbage, shredded**
**25g/1oz butter**
**4 tsp oil**
**1 small onion, peeled and very finely chopped**
**2 cloves garlic, peeled and crushed**
**3 tbsp Worcestershire sauce**

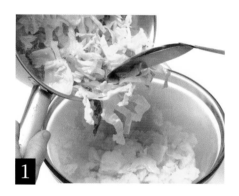

1 Preheat the oven to 190°C/375°F/Gas Mark 5. Cook the potatoes in a large pan of boiling water for 10–15 minutes or until tender. Drain thoroughly and mash. Cook the cabbage in a large pan of boiling water for 5–8 minutes or until just tender. Drain thoroughly and add to the mashed potato along with the butter, stirring well to mix.

2 In a small frying pan, heat the oil and add the onion and garlic. Cook for 3–4 minutes until softened. Add to the cabbage mixture along with any oil remaining in the pan. Add the Worcestershire sauce and stir well.

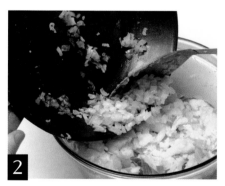

3 Divide the mixture into 4 (8) and place on a lightly greased baking sheet in rough piles, flattening slightly. Rough up a little with a fork. Place in the preheated oven and bake for 30–35 minutes, turning halfway through, until golden in places and starting to crisp. Serve.

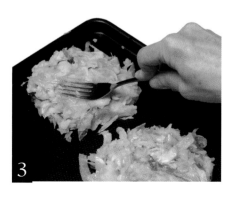

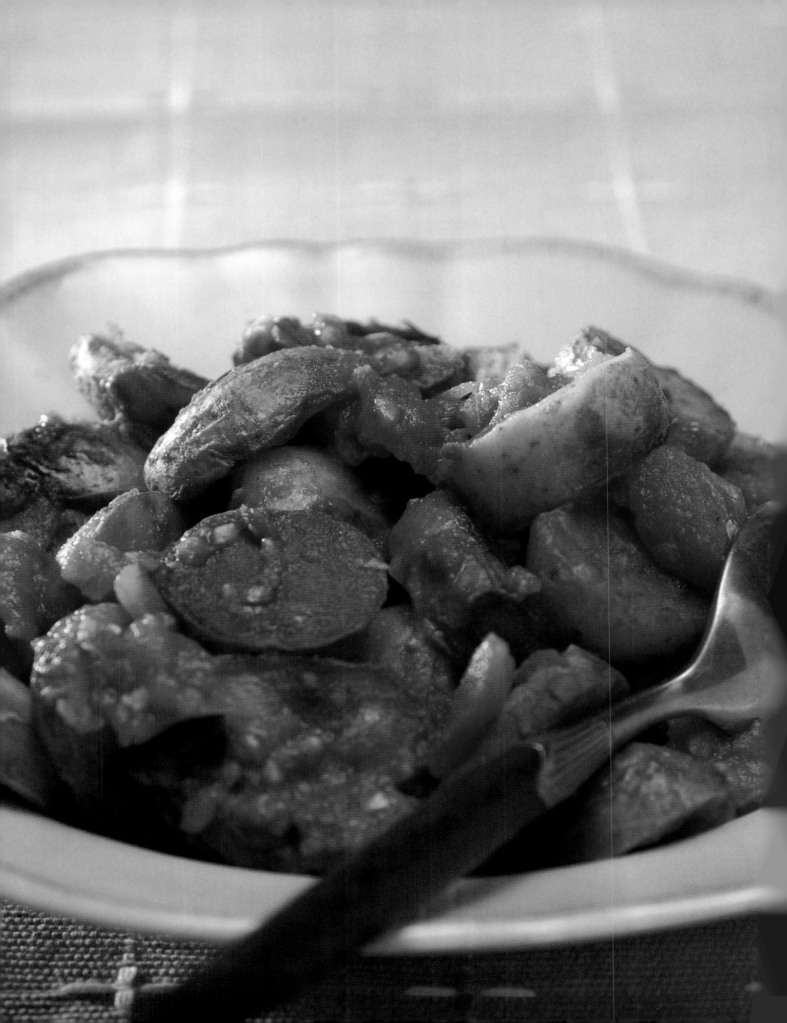

# Spiced Potatoes with Tomato

*vegetarian*

Potatoes are often cooked in a way that makes them fattening, but they don't have to be as this recipe shows.

### Serves 2

3 tomatoes
350g/12oz waxy potatoes, peeled
2 tsp olive oil
1 clove garlic, peeled and crushed
2 tsp smoked paprika

### Serves 4

6 tomatoes
700g/1½lb waxy potatoes, peeled
4 tsp olive oil
2 cloves garlic, peeled and crushed
4 tsp smoked paprika

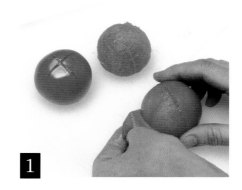

1 Cut a cross in the base of each tomato, cover with boiling water and leave for 1 minute. Remove from the water and peel, then chop and set to one side. Cut the potatoes into bite-size chunks. Bring a large pan of water to the boil. Add the potatoes and bring back to the boil. Reduce the heat a little and cover. Cook for 8 minutes and drain.

2 Heat the oil in a large frying pan and add the potatoes. Cook over a moderate heat stirring from time to time for about 10 minutes, until the potatoes start to turn golden in places.

3 Add the garlic and paprika and cook, stirring, for 1 minute.

4 Add the chopped tomatoes and continue to cook for a further 5 minutes, stirring from time to time. Remove from the heat and serve.

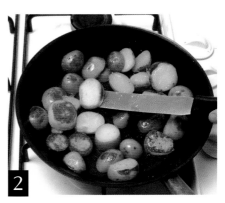

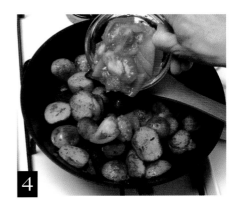

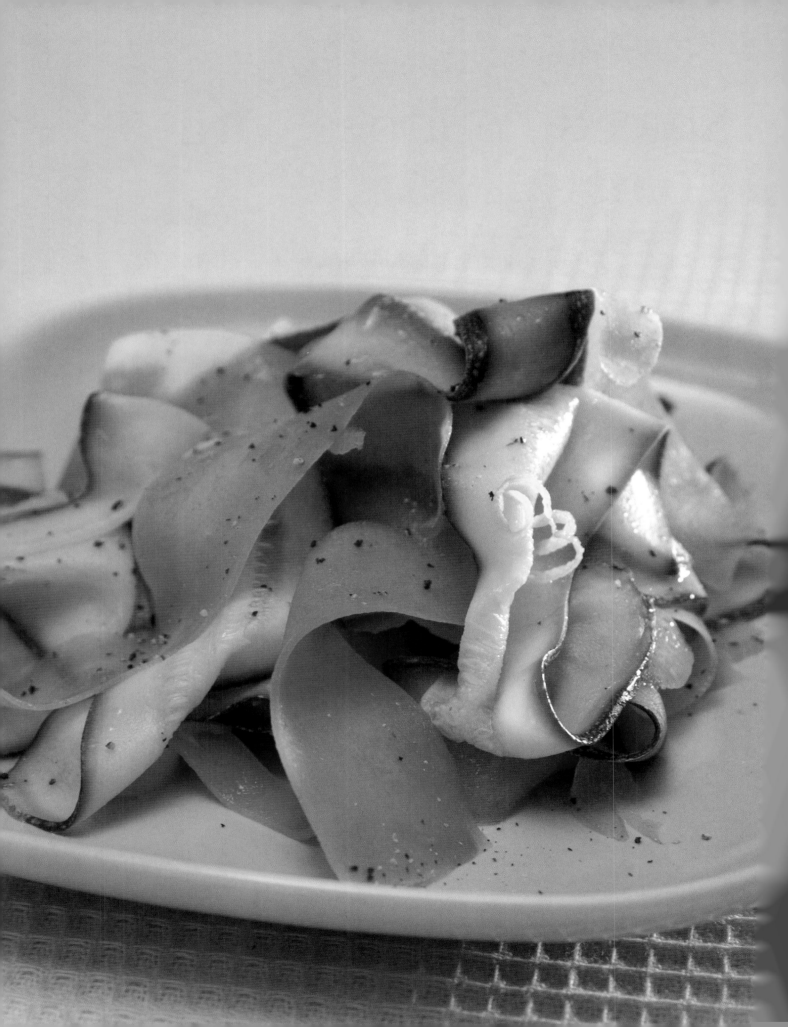

# Steamed Carrot & Courgette Strips

*Easy Entertaining*

By lightly steaming these vegetables, most of the nutrients are kept.

## Serves 2

**2 medium carrots, peeled**
**2 medium courgettes, trimmed**
**1 clove garlic, peeled and crushed**
**1 tbsp olive oil**
**½ lemon**
**freshly ground black pepper**

## Serves 4

**4 medium carrots, peeled**
**4 medium courgettes, trimmed**
**2 cloves garlic, peeled and crushed**
**2 tbsp olive oil**
**1 lemon**
**freshly ground black pepper**

1 Using a vegetable peeler, cut the carrot into ribbons.

2 Repeat with the courgette.

3 Bring a large saucepan of water to the boil and place a steamer over it. Place the prepared carrot and courgette in the steamer and cook for 3–4 minutes until piping hot and just tender.

4 In a small mixing bowl, whisk the garlic and olive oil together. Finely grate the zest from the lemon, squeeze the juice and add to the oil and garlic. Stir to combine.

5 Place in a serving dish and gently toss through the lemon and garlic oil. Season with freshly ground black pepper and serve.

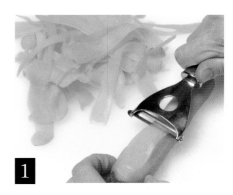

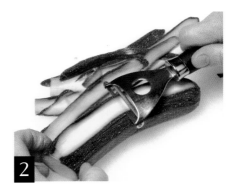

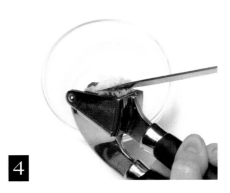

# Dry Curried Spinach

*vegetarian*

Turmeric has been found to be helpful in guarding against Alzheimer's disease.

## Serves 2

1 tbsp sunflower oil
1 small onion, peeled and
    sliced
1 clove garlic, peeled and
    crushed
1 tsp ground cumin
½ tsp turmeric
¼ tsp dried red chilli flakes
1 x 200g/7oz can tomatoes,
    chopped
150g/5oz spinach, washed
    and tough stalks
    removed
plain yoghurt to serve

## Serves 4

2 tbsp sunflower oil
1 onion, peeled and sliced
2 cloves garlic, peeled and
    crushed
2 tsp ground cumin
1 tsp turmeric
½ tsp dried red chilli flakes
1 x 400g/14oz can tomatoes,
    chopped
300g/10½oz spinach,
    washed and tough stalks
    removed
plain yoghurt to serve

1 Heat the oil in a large pan and cook the onion over a moderate heat until it becomes softened. Add the crushed garlic and cook for a further minute.

2 Stir in the spices and cook for 1–2 minutes. Pour over the tomatoes and bring gently to the boil. Reduce the heat to a gentle simmer and cook, uncovered, for 5–10 minutes until the mixture thickens.

3 Stir in the spinach and continue to cook until it wilts. Spoon over a little plain yoghurt and serve.

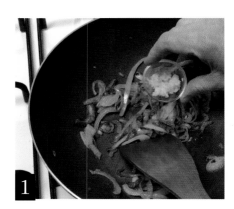

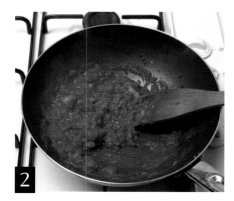

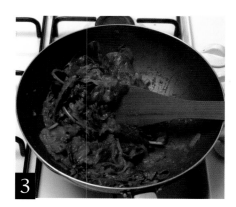

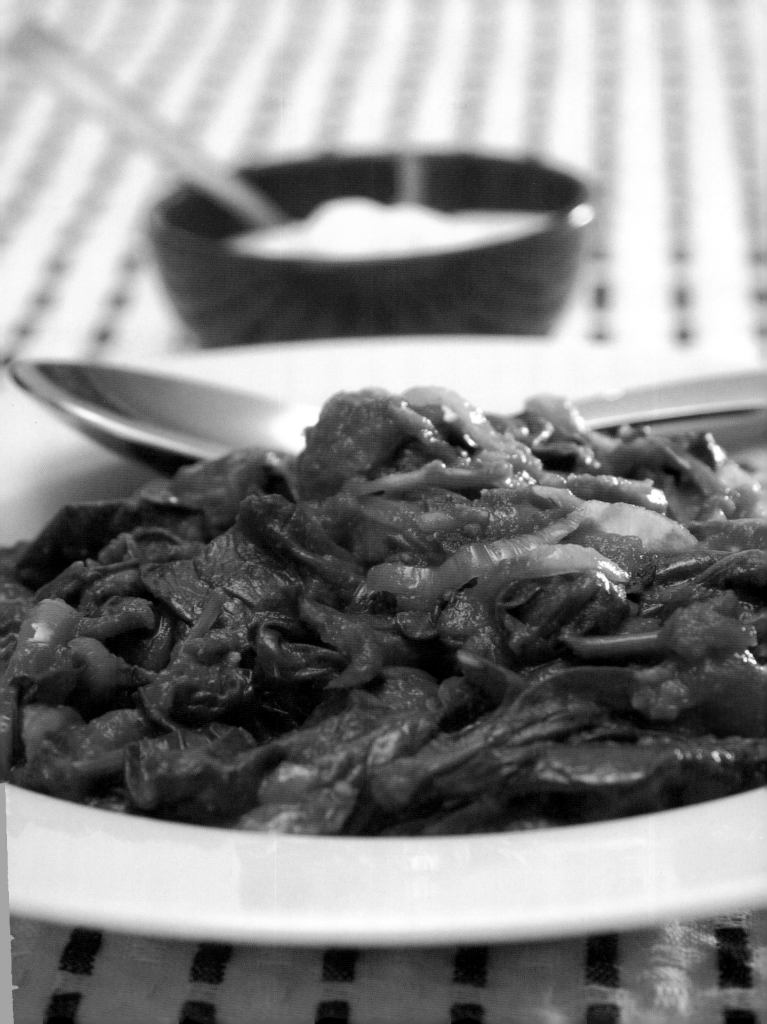

# Spiced Oven Jacket Chips

## *Children's Choice*

You can still have chips, but by cooking them this way the fat content is dramatically reduced.

### Serves 2

**400g/14oz potatoes,**
   **scrubbed**
**1 tbsp olive oil**
**½ tsp salt**
**½ tsp black pepper**
**pinch cayenne pepper**
**¼ tsp ground cumin**

### Serves 4

**800g/1lb 12oz potatoes,**
   **scrubbed**
**2 tbsp olive oil**
**1 tsp salt**
**1 tsp black pepper**
**¼ tsp cayenne pepper**
**½ tsp ground cumin**

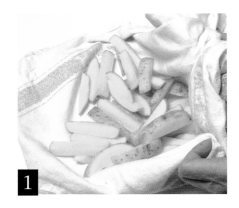

1. Preheat the oven to 200°C/400°F/Gas Mark 6. Cut the potatoes into chips and pat them dry with a clean tea towel. Place in a mixing bowl and drizzle over the olive oil, tossing well to mix. Spread in a single layer over a non-stick heavy-gauge baking tray. Alternatively line a heavy-gauge baking tray with baking parchment or silicone sheet.

2. Place in the preheated oven and cook for 15 minutes. In a small bowl, mix together the salt, black pepper, cayenne pepper and cumin.

3. Remove the chips from the oven, turn using a fish slice and sprinkle with the spice mixture. Return to the oven and cook for a further 15 minutes until golden and crisp. Serve.

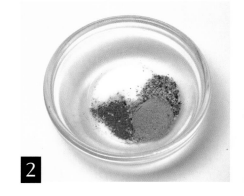

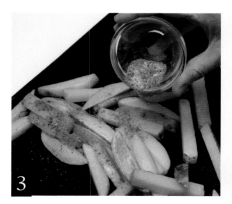

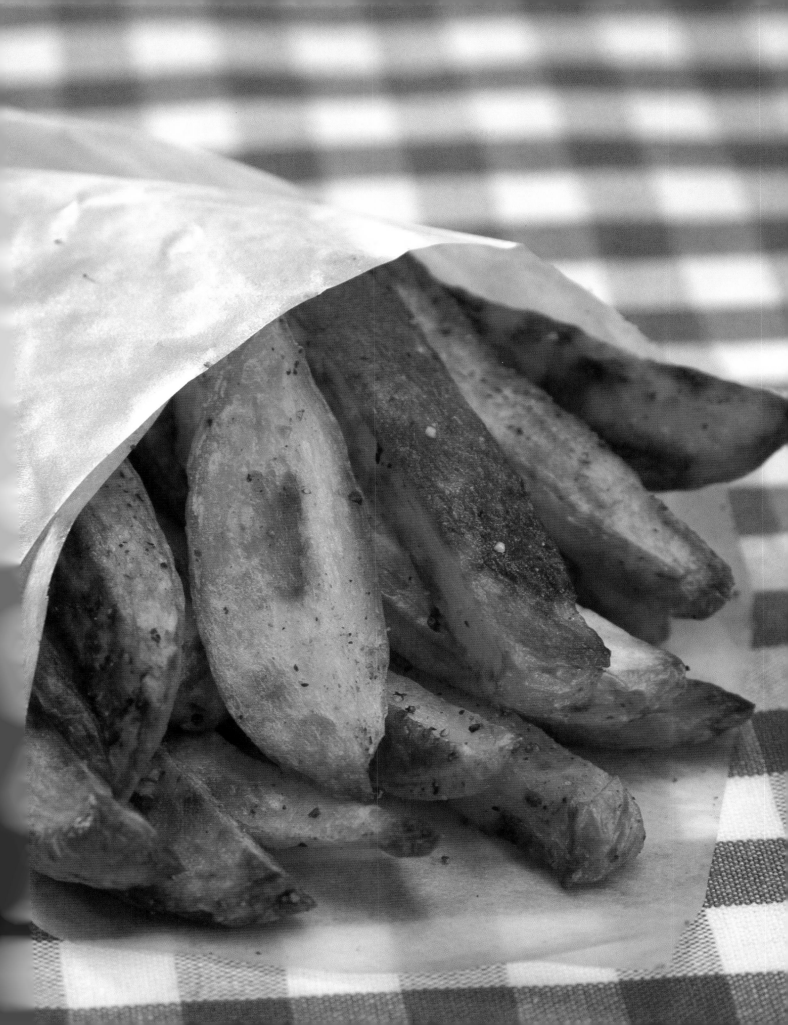

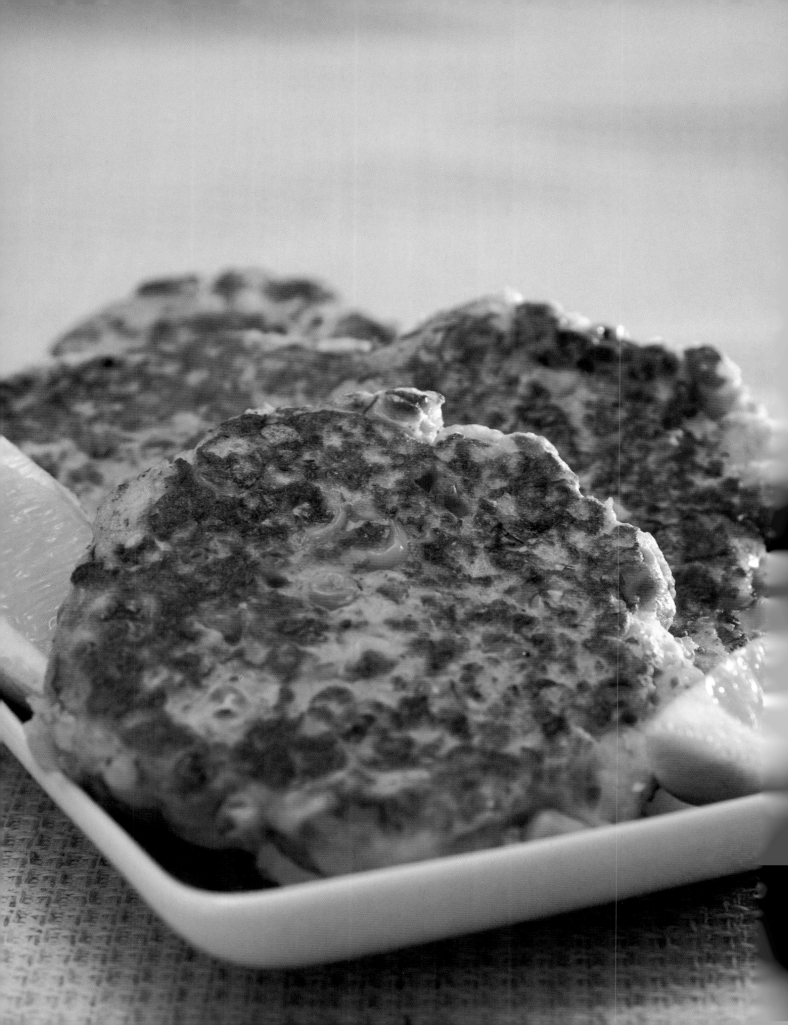

# Spiced Potato Cakes

## Children's Choice

Potato cakes with peas and sweetcorn are a simple way to get children to eat a few more vegetables in their diets.

### Serves 2

**300g/10½oz potatoes**
**15g/½oz flour**
**50g/ 2oz peas, cooked**
**75g/3oz sweetcorn**
**1 tsp curry powder**
**1 small clove garlic, peeled
and crushed**
**2 tbsp fresh coriander,
chopped**
**½ egg, beaten**
**oil for spraying**
**lemon wedges to serve**

### Serves 4

**600g/1lb 5oz potatoes**
**25g/1oz flour**
**100g/4oz peas, cooked**
**150g/5oz sweetcorn**
**2 tsp curry powder**
**1 clove garlic, peeled and
crushed**
**4 tbsp fresh coriander,
chopped**
**1 egg, beaten**
**oil for spraying**
**lemon wedges to serve**

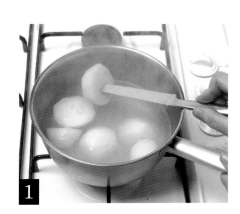

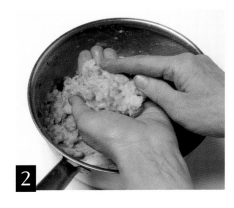

1 Peel the potatoes and cut into quarters. Place in a large saucepan of cold water and bring to the boil. Reduce the heat to a simmer and cook for approximately 12 minutes, or until the potatoes are tender when tested with the tip of a knife. Remove from the heat and drain thoroughly.

2 Mash the potatoes until smooth and no lumps remain. Add the flour, peas, sweetcorn, curry powder, garlic, coriander and egg and mix well. Using damp hands, divide the mixture into 4 (8) equal-sized pieces. Shape each piece into a ball and then flatten slightly.

3 Heat a non-stick frying pan over a moderate heat and spray lightly with a little oil. Cook each pattie for about 6–8 minutes or until golden and piping hot, turning halfway through. Serve with lemon wedges.

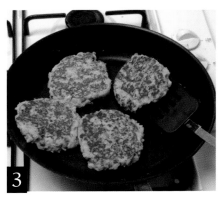

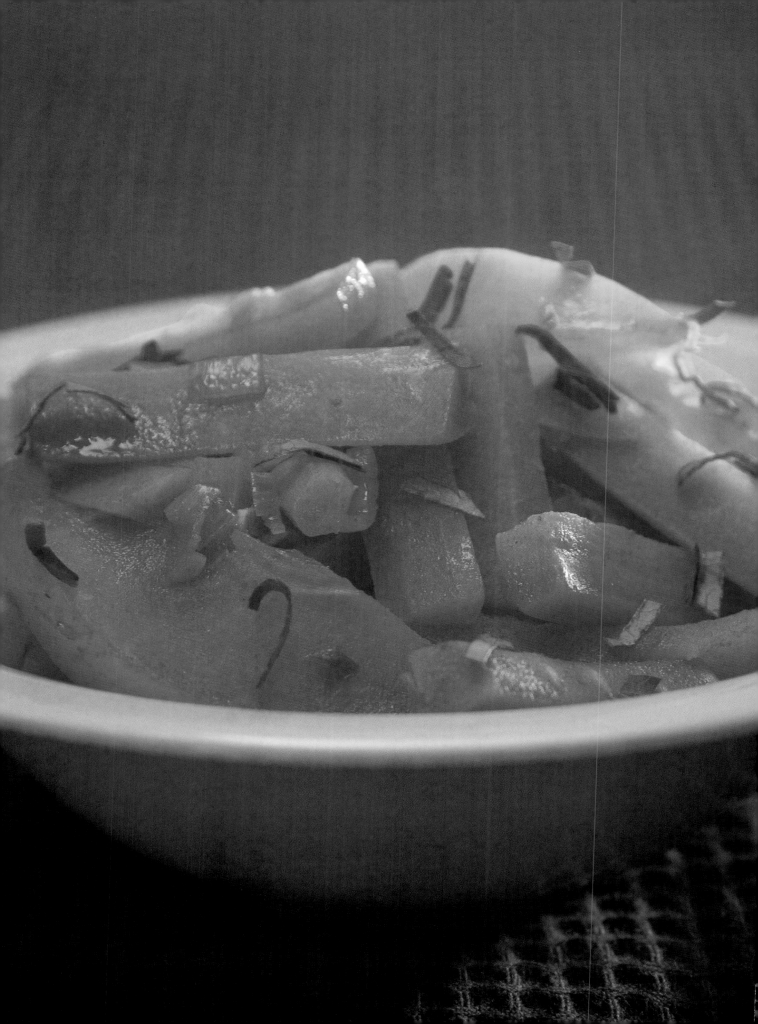

# Sweet & Spiced Carrots

*One Pot*

A simple dish that is a tasty accompaniment.

### Serves 2

**1 tbsp sunflower oil**
**2 shallots, peeled and**
**chopped**
**1 clove garlic, peeled and**
**finely chopped**
**1 tsp smoked paprika**
**350g/12oz carrots, peeled**
**and sliced into batons**
**1 eating apple, cored and**
**thinly sliced**
**100ml/3½fl oz apple juice**

### Serves 4

**2 tbsp sunflower oil**
**4 shallots, peeled and**
**chopped**
**2 cloves garlic, peeled and**
**finely chopped**
**2 tsp smoked paprika**
**700g/1½lb carrots, peeled**
**and sliced into batons**
**1 large eating apple, cored**
**and thinly sliced**
**200ml/7fl oz apple juice**

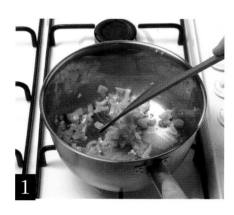

1 In a large saucepan with a well-fitting lid, heat the oil over a moderate heat. Add the shallots and garlic and cook until softened.

2 Add the smoked paprika and cook for 1 minute, stirring. Stir in the carrots and apple, mixing well to coat in the shallots and spiced oil and cook for 2–3 minutes.

3 Pour over the apple juice and bring gently to the boil. Reduce the heat to a gentle simmer and cover the pan. Cook for 20 minutes until the carrots are tender. Serve.

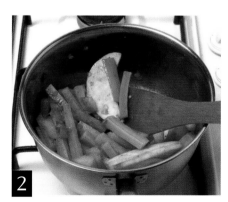

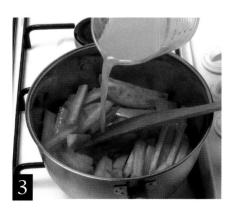

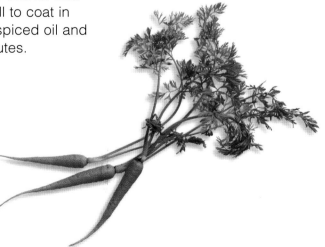

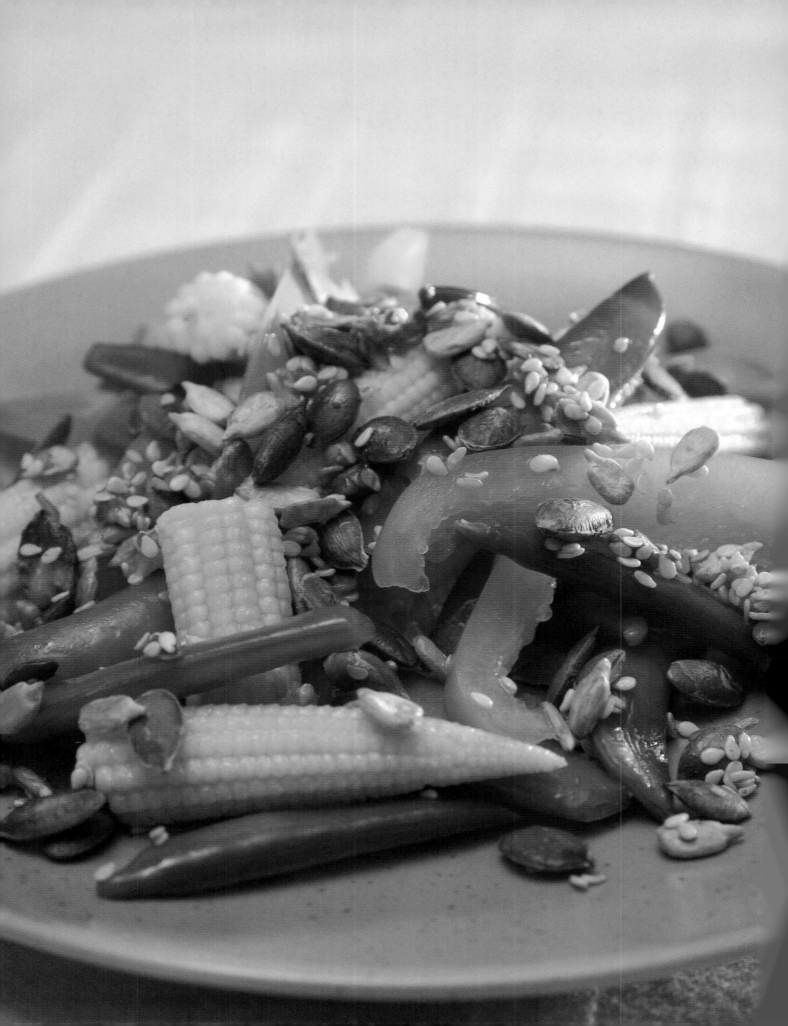

# Seeded Salad

## Children's Choice

Including seeds in this salad is not only tasty but also provides vitamin E, fibre, protein and unsaturated fats.

### Serves 2

**1 tbsp sesame seeds**
**2 tbsp pumpkin seeds**
**1 tbsp sunflower seeds**
**1 tsp dark soy sauce**
**1 small clove garlic, peeled and crushed**
**pinch cayenne pepper**
**1 orange pepper**
**100g/4oz sugar snaps**
**6 baby corn, halved**
**1cm/½in fresh ginger, peeled and finely grated**
**1 tsp sesame oil**
**1 tsp honey**
**1 tbsp lemon juice**

### Serves 4

**2 tbsp sesame seeds**
**4 tbsp pumpkin seeds**
**2 tbsp sunflower seeds**
**2 tsp dark soy sauce**
**1 clove garlic, peeled and crushed**
**¼ tsp cayenne pepper**
**2 orange peppers**
**200g/7oz sugar snaps**
**12 baby corn, halved**
**2.5cm/1in fresh ginger, peeled and finely grated**
**2 tsp sesame oil**
**2 tsp honey**
**2 tbsp lemon juice**

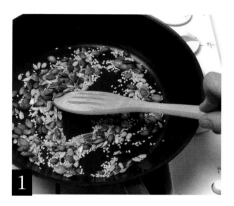

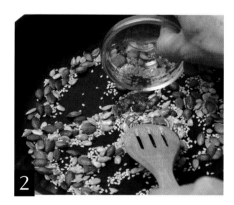

1 Mix the seeds together and cook in a small non-stick frying pan until lightly toasted.

2 Remove from the heat. Add the soy sauce, garlic and cayenne pepper and mix well. Set to one side to cool.

3 Deseed the pepper and cut into thin strips, then place in a bowl. Bring a saucepan of water to the boil and cook the sugar snaps and baby corn for 3 minutes at a rolling boil. Drain, then cover with cold water to stop them cooking further.

4 Mix the ginger, sesame oil, honey and lemon juice together in a small bowl. Drain the cooled sugar snaps and baby corn and add to the pepper strips. Drizzle over the ginger and lemon dressing and toss well to mix. Sprinkle over the toasted seeds to serve.

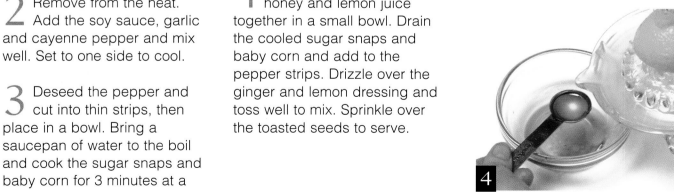

# Pear, Walnut & Watercress Salad

*Easy Entertaining*

The sweetness of the pear goes beautifully with the pepperiness of the watercress.

## Serves 2

1 tbsp walnut oil
1 tbsp cider vinegar
40g/1½oz walnuts, roughly
  chopped
1 ripe pear
75g/3oz watercress

## Serves 4

2 tbsp walnut oil
2 tbsp cider vinegar
75g/3oz walnuts, roughly
  chopped
2 ripe pears
150g/5oz watercress

1 Preheat the grill to high. In a small mixing bowl beat the walnut oil and vinegar together.

2 Place a small frying pan over a moderate heat and dry fry the walnuts, tossing them from time to time, until they smell toasted and fragrant. Remove from the pan or they will continue to cook and possibly burn, and set to one side.

3 Core the pear and cut into thin wedges. Brush the cut edges with a little of the oil and vinegar mixture.

4 Place under the hot grill for 3–4 minutes each side or until they start to turn golden in places. Remove from the heat.

5 Place the watercress in a serving bowl and top with the cooked pear wedges. Drizzle over the remaining oil and vinegar and scatter over the toasted walnuts. Serve.

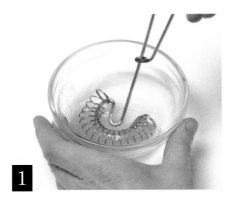

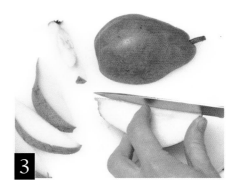

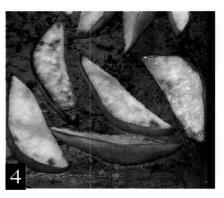

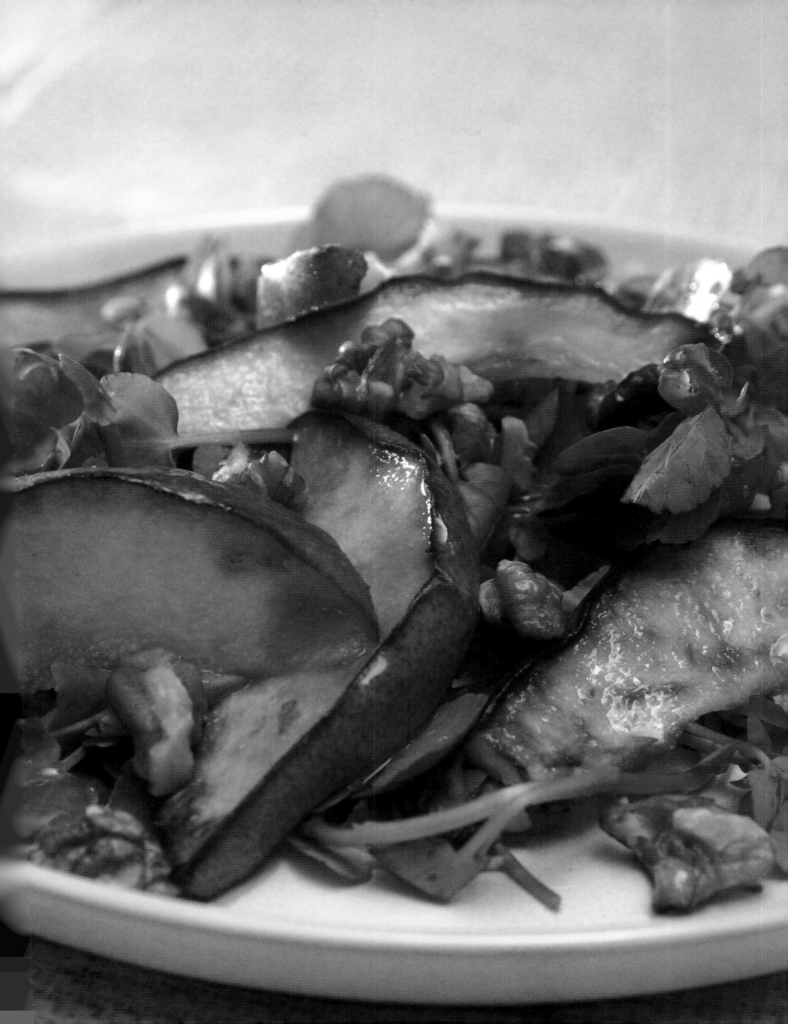

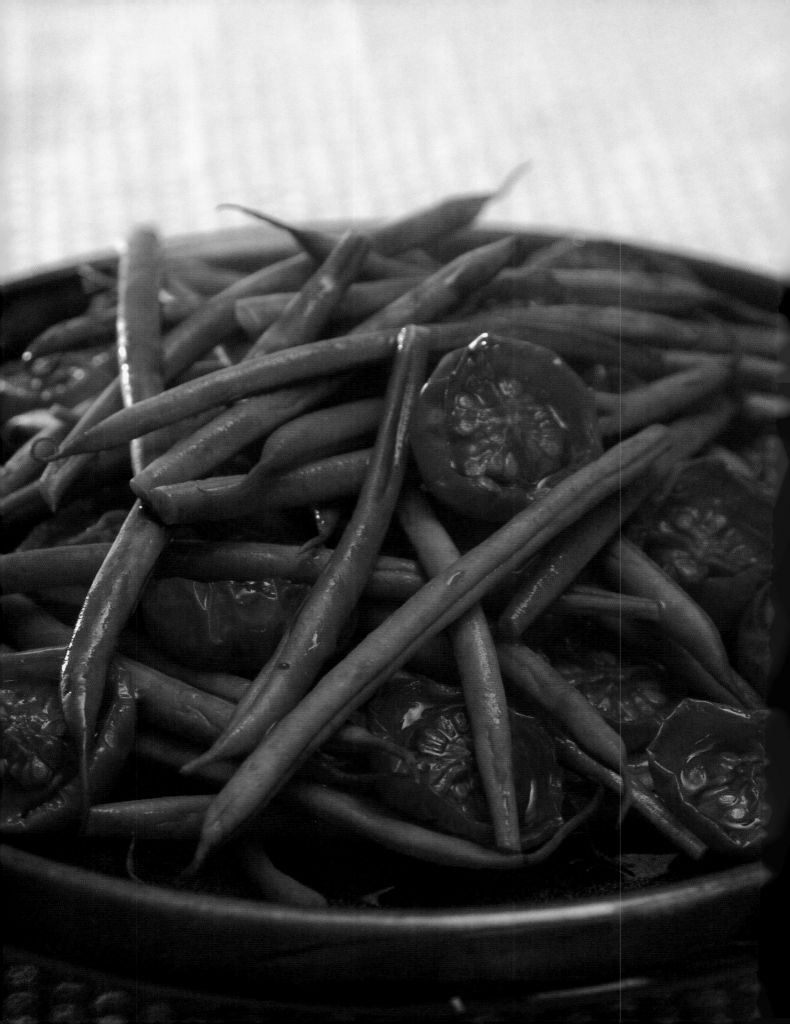

# Warm Tomato & Green Bean Salad

*vegetarian*

By cooking the tomatoes in this way the flavour becomes much more intense.

## Serves 2

**250g/9oz cherry tomatoes, halved**
**225g/8oz fine green beans, trimmed**
**1 tbsp balsamic vinegar**
**1 tbsp olive oil**
**1 tbsp basil leaves shredded**
**freshly ground black pepper**

## Serves 4

**500g/1lb 2oz cherry tomatoes, halved**
**450g/1lb fine green beans, trimmed**
**2 tbsp balsamic vinegar**
**2 tbsp olive oil**
**2 tbsp basil leaves shredded**
**freshly ground black pepper**

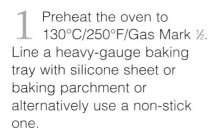

1 Preheat the oven to 130°C/250°F/Gas Mark ½. Line a heavy-gauge baking tray with silicone sheet or baking parchment or alternatively use a non-stick one.

2 Arrange the tomatoes in a single layer over the prepared baking sheet and cook in the preheated oven for 2½–3 hours until the tomatoes are semi dried.

3 About ten minutes before the tomatoes are ready, bring a large saucepan of water to the boil and then cook the beans for 3–4 minutes until just tender but still with a little bite. Drain.

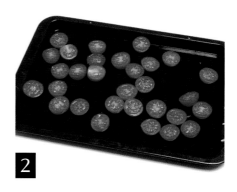

4 Toss the beans, balsamic vinegar and oil through the semi-dried tomatoes and return to the oven for 5 minutes. Sprinkle with shredded basil leaves, season with freshly ground black pepper and serve.

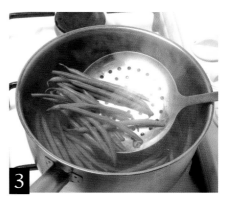

# Orange & Beetroot Salad

*Quick and Easy*

Beetroots are a good source of folate, which is important for healthy cells.

**Serves 2**

2 oranges
2 cooked beetroot
40g/1½oz feta cheese
50g/2oz mixed sprouted
   beans
50g/2oz watercress

**Serves 4**

4 oranges
4 cooked beetroot
75g/3oz feta cheese
100g/4oz mixed sprouted
   beans
100g/4oz watercress

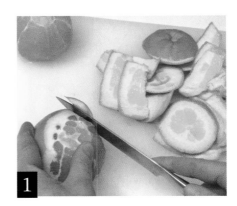

1 To peel the oranges first cut a slice from the top and bottom of each one. Now slice away the skin and pith by cutting from top to bottom, rotating the orange as you do so.

2 Cut the flesh into thin slices and place in a mixing bowl along with any juices that may have collected on the chopping board.

3 Thinly slice the beetroot, add to the oranges and toss lightly to mix.

4 Crumble over the feta cheese and add the mixed bean sprouts. Toss lightly to mix. Divide the watercress between the serving plates and top with the beetroot and orange mixture. Serve.

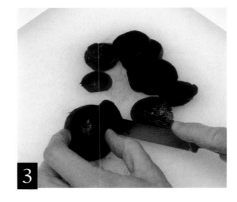

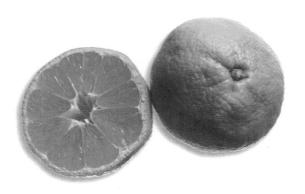

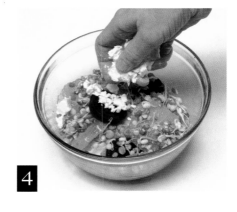

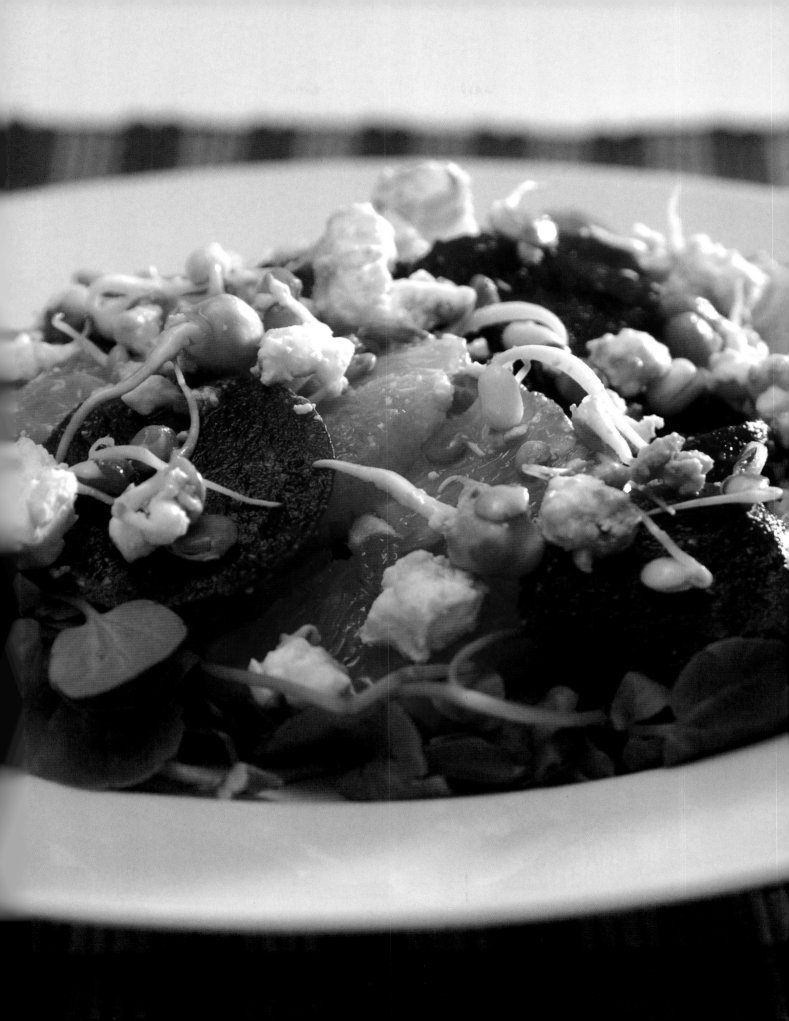

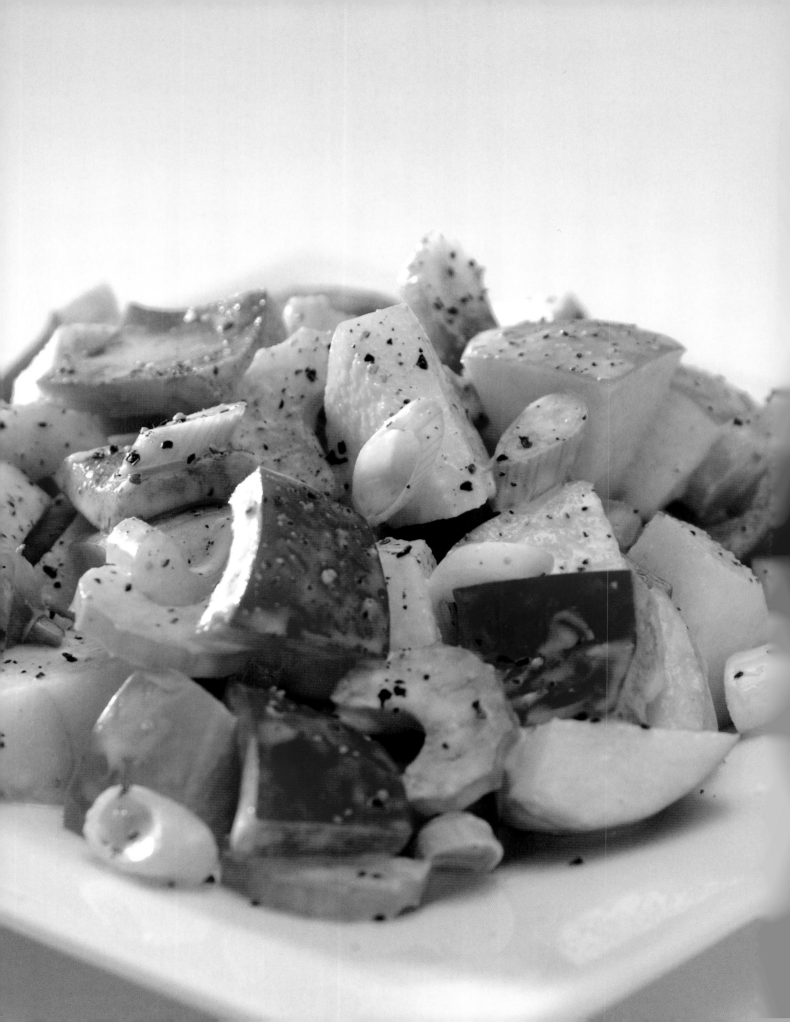

# Apple & Pepper Salad

*Quick and Easy*

A crunchy colourful salad, full of vitamin C.

**Serves 2**

2 green apples
2 tsp lemon juice
1 small red pepper
2 sticks celery
2 spring onions
1 tbsp mayonnaise
1 tbsp plain yoghurt
black pepper to serve

**Serves 4**

4 green apples
4 tsp lemon juice
1 red pepper
4 sticks celery
4 spring onions
2 tbsp mayonnaise
2 tbsp plain yoghurt
black pepper to serve

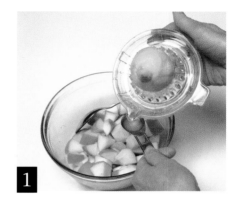

1 Core the apples, cut into bite-size pieces and place in a mixing bowl with the lemon juice. Toss well to coat.

2 Halve and deseed the pepper and cut into bite-size chunks. Add to the apple pieces.

3 Thinly slice the celery and spring onions and add to the apple and pepper.

4 Mix the mayonnaise and yoghurt together with 1 (2) tbsp cold water. Pour over the prepared salad and toss well to mix. Season with a little black pepper and serve.

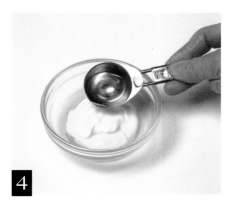

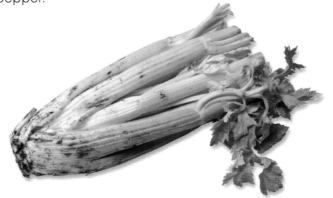

# Coriander Coleslaw

*Quick and Easy*

Eating vegetables raw is often a good way to tempt reluctant children, as they enjoy the crunchiness.

## Serves 2

**2 slices Parma ham**
**1 small clove garlic, peeled and crushed**
**1 tbsp olive oil**
**½ tbsp balsamic vinegar**
**½ tsp Dijon mustard**
**¼ tsp caster sugar**
**175g/6oz white cabbage**
**125g/4½oz carrots, peeled**
**½ small red onion, peeled**
**3 tbsp fresh coriander, chopped**

## Serves 4

**4 slices Parma ham**
**1 clove garlic, peeled and crushed**
**2 tbsp olive oil**
**1 tbsp balsamic vinegar**
**1 tsp Dijon mustard**
**½ tsp caster sugar**
**350g/12oz white cabbage**
**250g/9oz carrots, peeled**
**1 small red onion, peeled**
**6 tbsp fresh coriander, chopped**

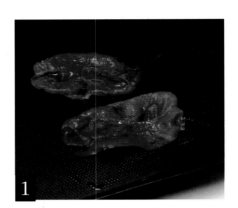

1 Preheat the grill to high and cook the Parma ham until golden and crisp. Remove from the heat and allow to cool.

2 Place the crushed garlic, olive oil, balsamic vinegar, Dijon mustard and sugar in a mixing bowl and whisk until fully combined.

3 Finely shred the white cabbage and coarsely grate the carrot into a large mixing bowl. Finely slice the red onion and toss through the cabbage and carrot to mix.

4 Drizzle over the dressing, add the coriander and mix well. Break the Parma ham into small pieces and scatter over the top of the coleslaw to serve.

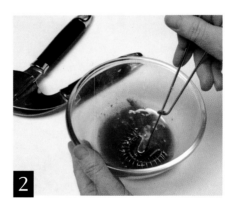

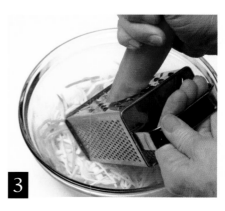

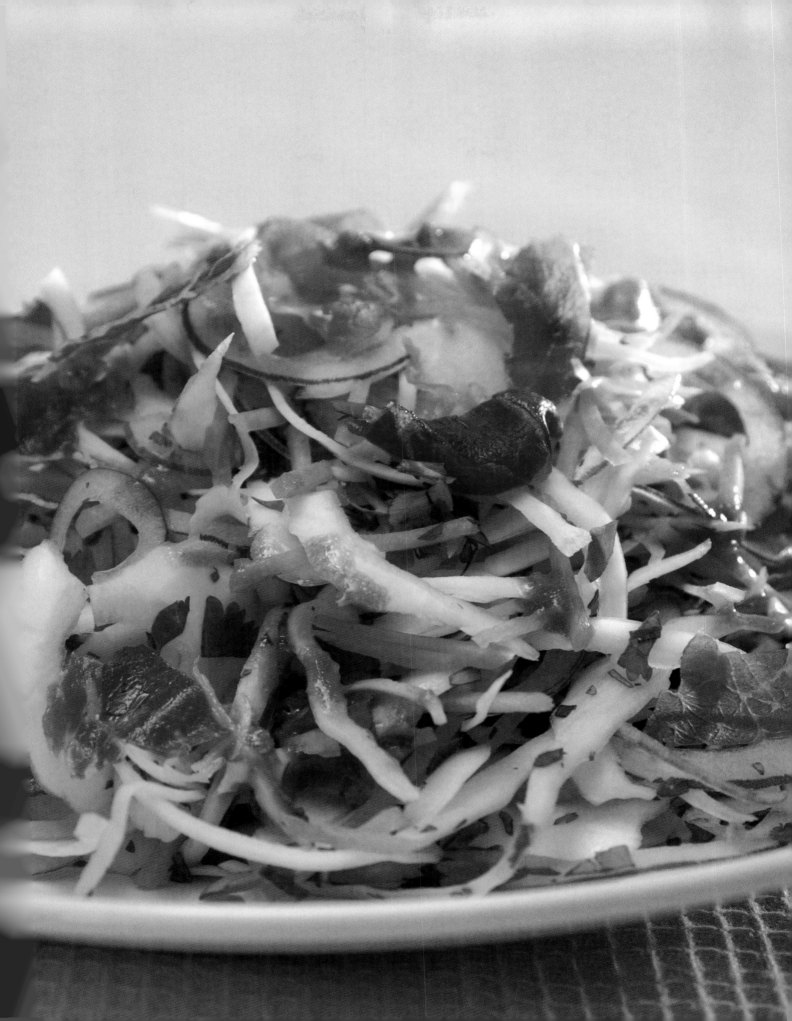

# Lentil Rice Salad

*vegetarian*

Lentils are helpful in reducing cholesterol levels as well as being low in fat, high in fibre and a good source of protein.

### Serves 2

50g/2oz Puy lentils
75g/3oz basmati rice
1 onion, peeled and thinly
   sliced
½ tbsp sunflower oil
½ tsp cumin seeds
1½ tbsp fresh parsley,
   chopped
freshly ground black pepper

### Serves 4

100g/4oz Puy lentils
150g/5oz basmati rice
1 large onion, peeled and
   thinly sliced
1 tbsp sunflower oil
1 tsp cumin seeds
3 tbsp fresh parsley,
   chopped
freshly ground black pepper

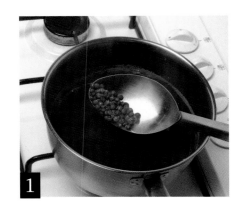

1 Place the lentils in a saucepan and cover with plenty of cold water. Bring to the boil and reduce the heat to a gentle simmer. Cook until the lentils are tender. Drain and set to one side.

2 Cook the basmati rice according to the packet instructions, then drain and toss through the cooked lentils.

3 Heat the oil in a large frying pan and cook the onion until it is softened. Add the cumin seeds and 1½ (3) tbsp of water and continue to cook until the onions are golden.

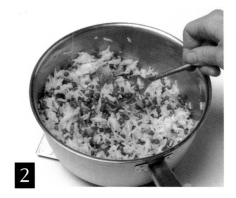

4 Add the contents of the frying pan to the cooked lentils and rice, stirring well to mix. Toss through the chopped parsley and season lightly with black pepper. Serve.

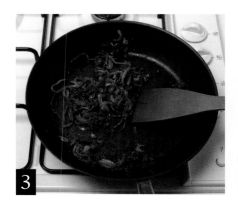

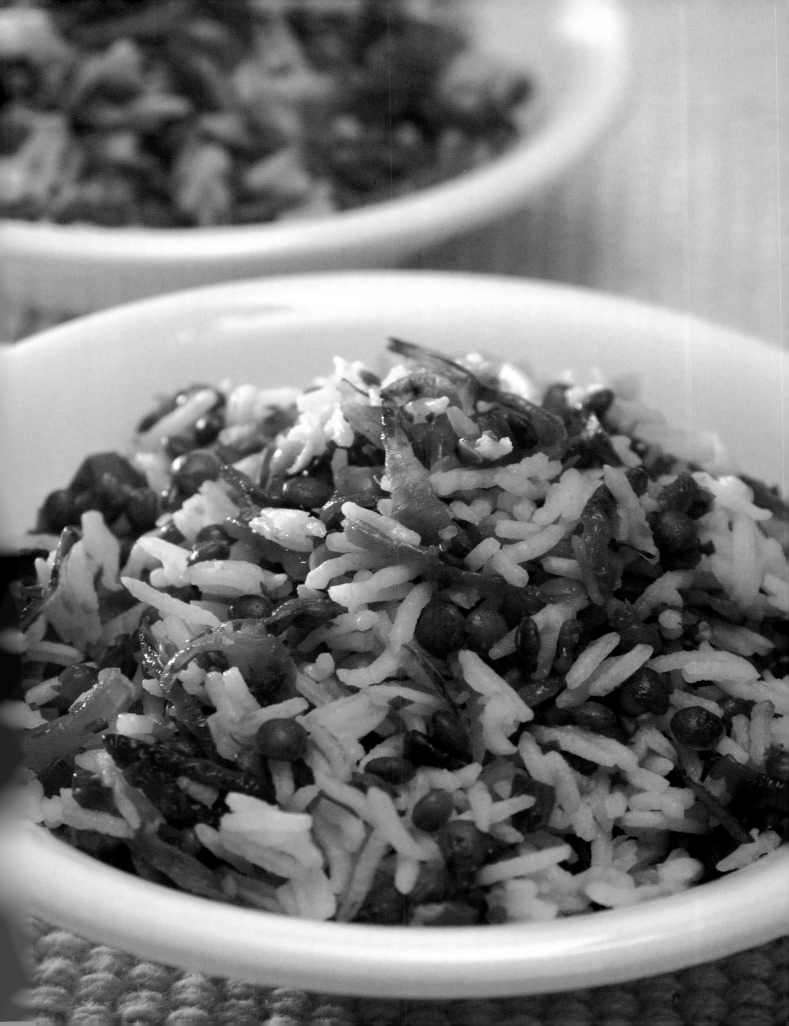

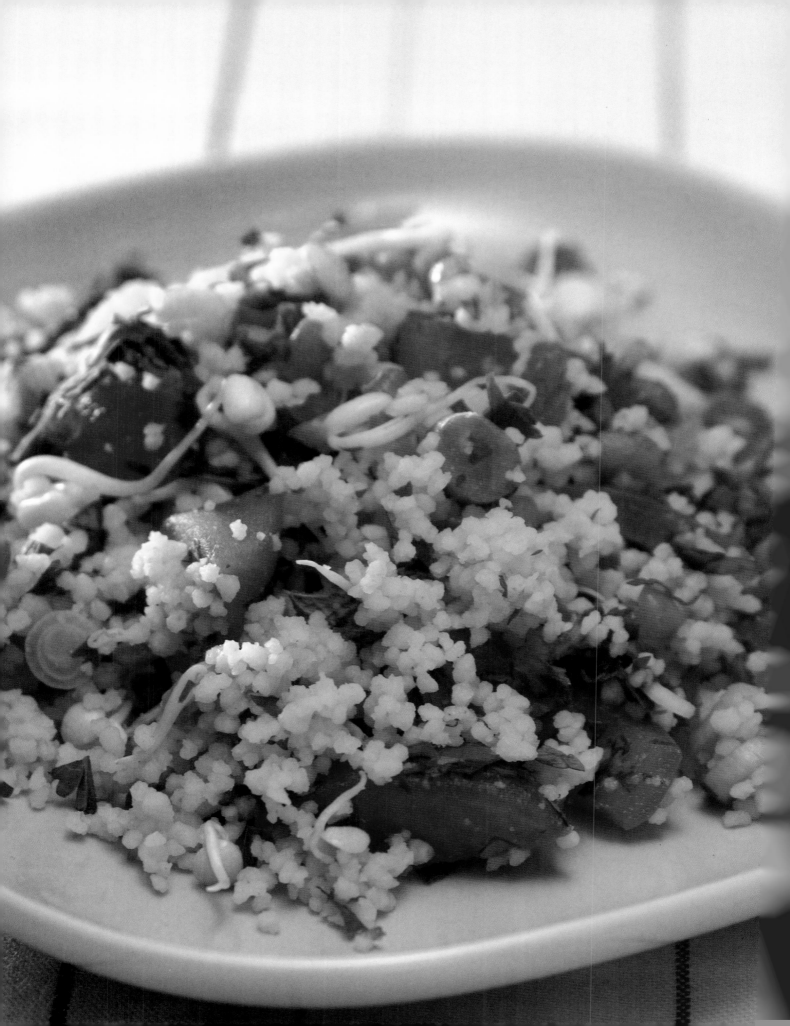

# Salsa & Bean Couscous

*Quick and Easy*

Bean sprouts are packed full of vitamin C and give a tasty crunch to this simple salad.

## Serves 2

**75g/3oz couscous**
**¼ vegetable stock cube**
**2 tomatoes**
**3 spring onions, finely sliced**
**1 small clove garlic, peeled**
    **and finely chopped**
**½ green chilli, thinly sliced**
**4 tbsp fresh coriander,**
    **chopped**
**pinch sugar**
**1 tbsp fresh lime juice**
**2 tbsp fresh mint, chopped**
**50g/2oz mixed bean sprouts**

## Serves 4

**175g/6oz couscous**
**½ vegetable stock cube**
**4 tomatoes**
**6 spring onions, finely sliced**
**1 clove garlic, peeled and**
    **finely chopped**
**1 green chilli, thinly sliced**
**8 tbsp fresh coriander,**
    **chopped**
**¼ tsp sugar**
**2 tbsp fresh lime juice**
**4 tbsp fresh mint, chopped**
**100g/4oz mixed bean sprouts**

1 Place the couscous in a large bowl. Dissolve the stock cube in 125ml/4fl oz (250ml/9fl oz) boiling water. Pour over the couscous and stir once. Cover with cling film and set to one side to soak for 10–15 minutes.

2 Using a sharp knife, cut a cross in the base of each tomato. Place in a bowl and cover with boiling water. Leave for 1 minute, remove from the water, peel and roughly chop.

3 Place the chopped tomatoes in a bowl with the spring onions, garlic, chilli, coriander, sugar and lime juice. Mix well and set to one side for 5 minutes.

4 Fork through the couscous to separate the grains. Add the mint and stir to mix. Lightly fold through the tomato salsa and mixed bean sprouts to serve.

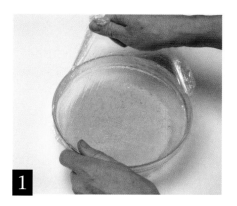

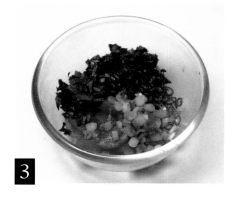

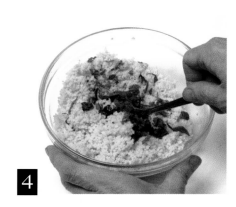

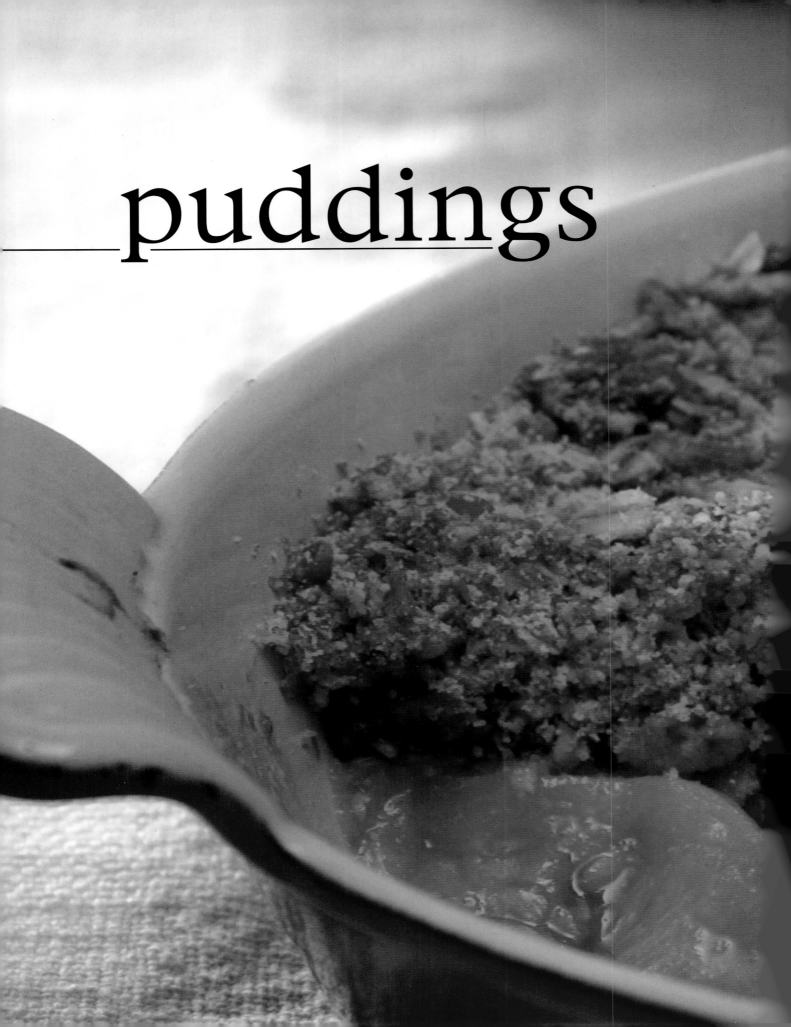

# puddings

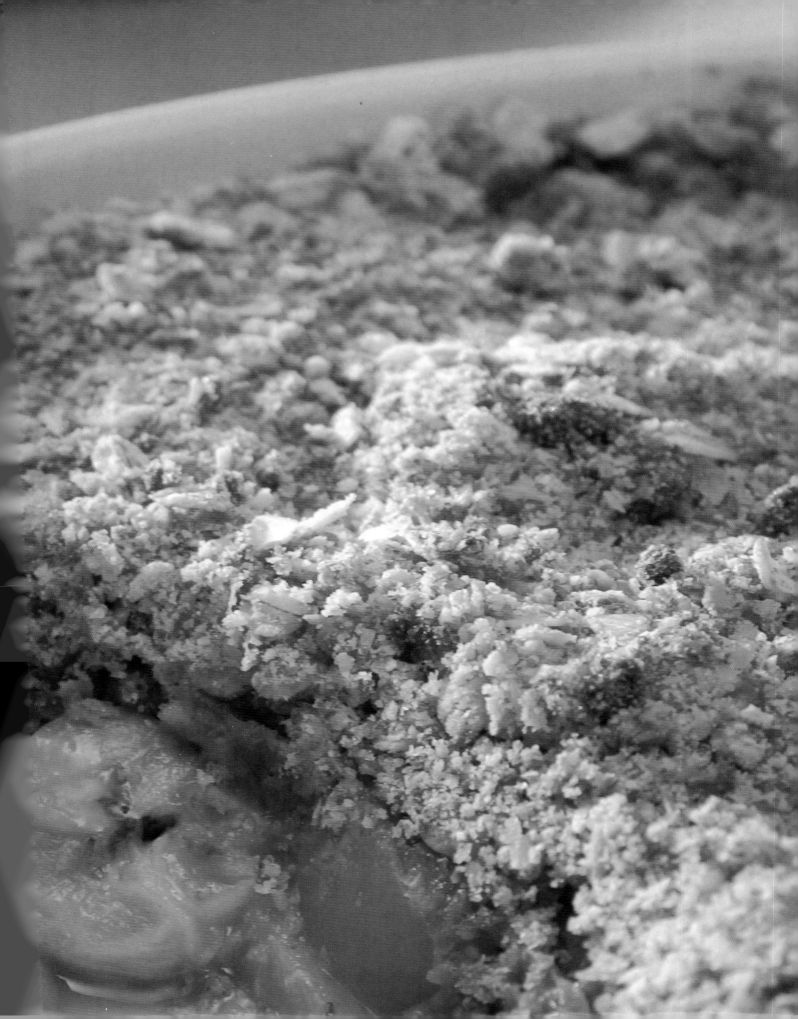

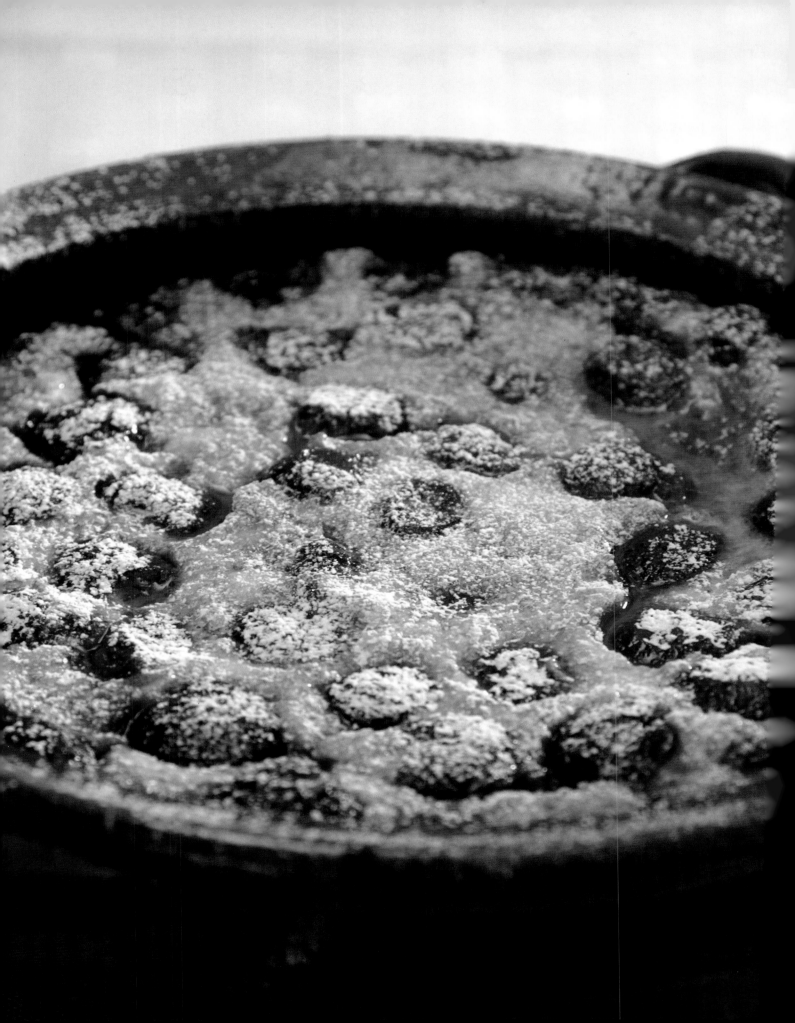

# Cherry Clafouti

## Easy Entertaining

Cherries contain potassium, which is helpful if you suffer from high blood pressure.

### Serves 4-6

**2 x 425g/15oz cans of cherries in juice, drained thoroughly**
**50g/2oz plain flour**
**100g/4oz caster sugar**
**15g/½oz butter, melted**
**200ml/7fl oz semi-skimmed milk**
**1 tsp vanilla essence**
**4 eggs, beaten**
**icing sugar for dusting**

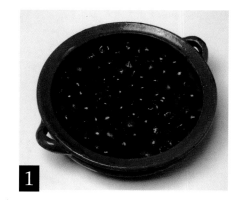

1 Preheat the oven to 190°C/375°F/Gas Mark 5. Lightly oil a shallow oven-proof dish and scatter the cherries over the base.

2 Sift the flour into a mixing bowl and add the sugar. Stir to mix, then make a well in the centre.

3 Beat the melted butter, milk, vanilla essence and eggs together. Pour this mixture into the flour and sugar and stir until it is smooth and all the flour has been incorporated.

4 Pour the batter over the cherries and bake in the preheated oven for 40 minutes until risen and golden. Allow to stand for 5 minutes. Dust with a little icing sugar before serving.

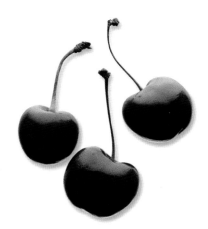

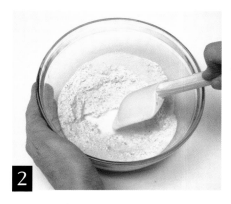

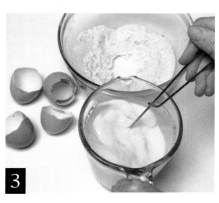

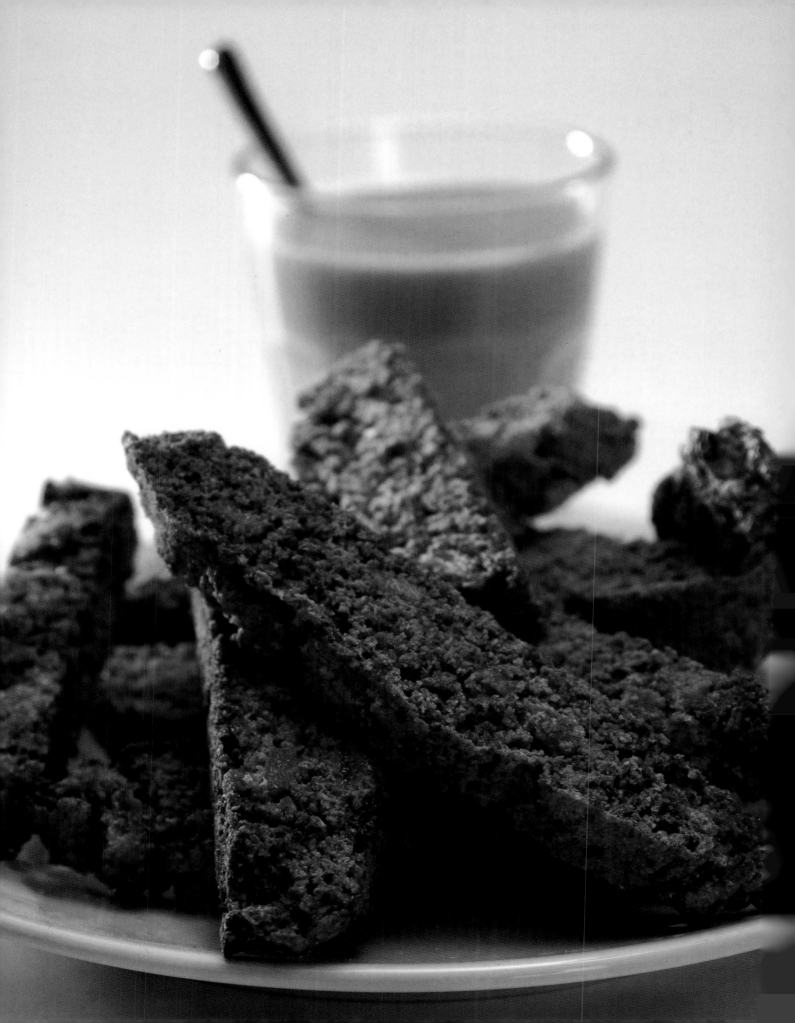

# Chocolate & Apricot Biscotti

*Easy Entertaining*

Dried apricots are not only a good source of fibre, but they also contain iron and potassium.

## Makes about 18

- **50g/2oz dark chocolate**
- **1 tbsp cocoa**
- **100g/4oz soft brown sugar**
- **100g/4oz wholemeal self-raising flour**
- **¼ tsp baking powder**
- **1 egg, beaten**
- **100g/4oz dried ready-to-eat apricots**

1 Preheat the oven to 180°C/350°F/Gas Mark 4. Roughly chop the chocolate and place in a food processor or blender with the cocoa and soft brown sugar. Process until the chocolate is finely chopped.

2 Tip the finely chopped chocolate mixture into a mixing bowl. Add the self-raising flour and baking powder and stir.

3 Add enough beaten egg to form a stiff dough and knead briefly. Now add the apricots and mix again.

4 Roughly shape the mixture into a log about 5cm/2in thick and place on a non-stick baking tray. Alternatively you can use a baking tray lined with silicone or baking parchment. Bake in the preheated oven for 25 minutes.

5 Remove from the oven and reduce the temperature to 140°C/275°F/ Gas Mark 1. Allow the log to cool for about 15 minutes.

6 Using a serrated knife, slice the log on the diagonal into 1cm/⅓in thick slices. Lay each slice back on the baking tray and return to the oven for a further 20 minutes, turning halfway through. Cool on a wire rack and store in an airtight container. Perfect served with dessert wine or coffee for dunking.

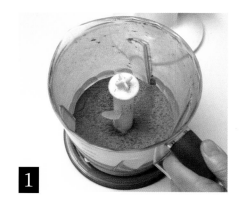

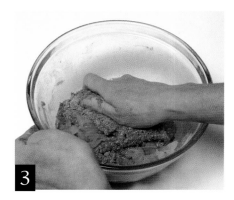

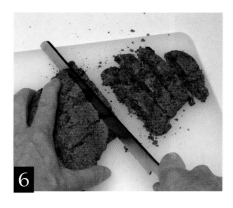

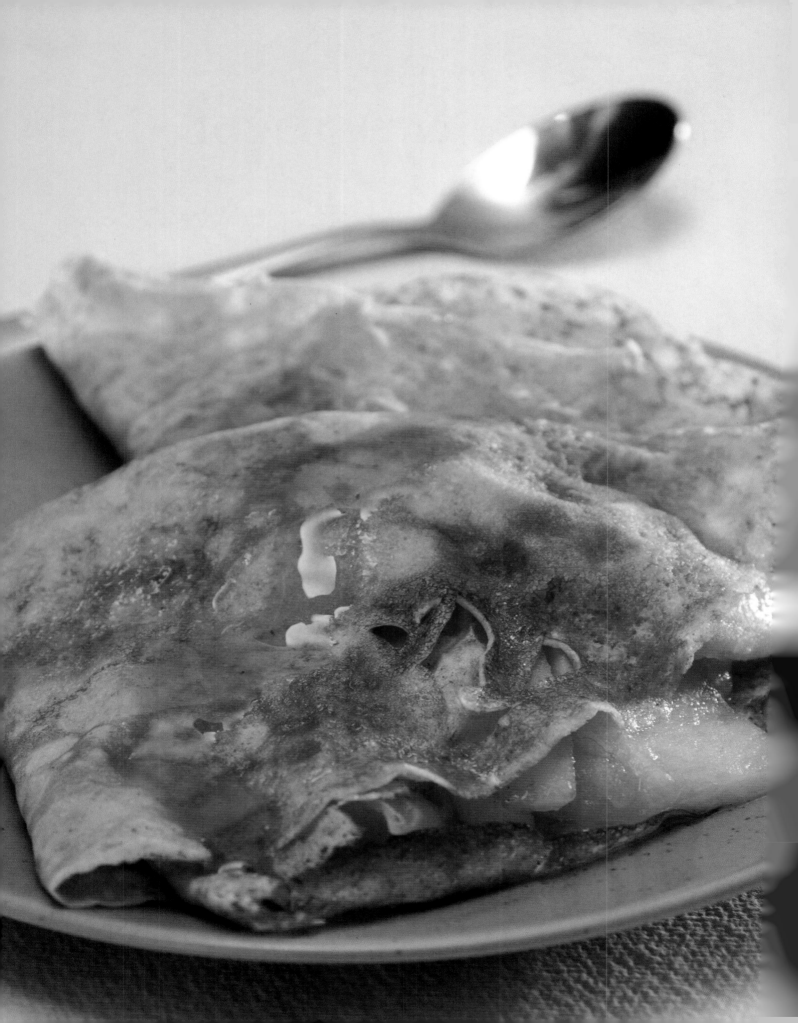

# Pancakes with Apples & Maple Syrup

*Children's Choice*

Pancakes are always a hit. Here they are teamed with apples, which are full of fibre and vitamin C.

### Serves 2

300g/10½oz apples, peeled,
   cored and sliced
1½ tbsp maple syrup
50g/2oz plain flour
½ egg, beaten
150ml/¼pt semi-skimmed
   milk
7g/¼oz butter

### Serves 4

600g/1lb 5oz apples, peeled,
   cored and sliced
3 tbsp maple syrup
100g/4oz plain flour
1 egg, beaten
300ml/½pt semi-skimmed
   milk
15g/½oz butter

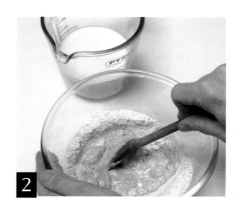

1 Place the sliced apples in a saucepan with 4 (8) tbsp cold water and 1 (2) tbsp of the maple syrup. Bring gently to the boil, reduce the heat to a gentle simmer. Cover with a well-fitting lid and cook, shaking the pan from time to time, for 20 minutes. Remove the pan from the heat and set to one side, still covered.

2 To make the pancake batter, sift the flour into a mixing bowl and make a well in the centre. Pour the beaten egg and a little milk into the well and stir, gradually drawing in the flour from around the edges. Add the rest of the milk and continue until all the flour has been incorporated and the mixture is smooth.

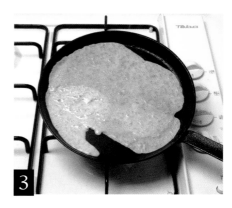

3 Heat the butter in a frying pan. Add the melted butter to the batter and stir to mix. Place the pan over a high heat and pour in enough batter to thinly coat the base, tipping the pan back and forth to cover it evenly. Cook for 1–2 minutes or until the pancake is golden. Turn and cook the other side until golden. Turn onto a plate and keep warm while you repeat the process, until all the batter has been used.

4 To serve, divide the stewed apple between the pancakes and fold to cover. Serve two stuffed pancakes per person. Drizzle the remaining maple syrup over the pancakes and serve.

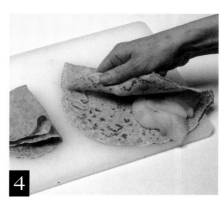

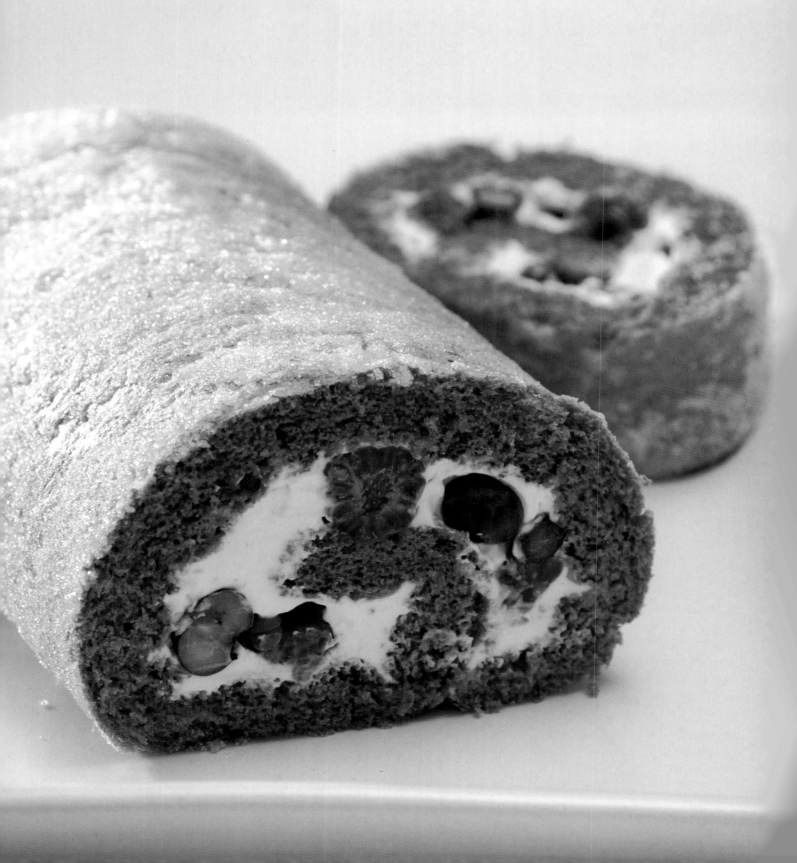

# Berry Roulade

*Easy Entertaining*

Low fat and very delicious, fill this roulade with your own choice of soft fruits if you wish.

*Serves 6*

**3 medium eggs**
**75g/3oz caster sugar, plus a little for sprinkling**
**60g/2½oz plain flour, sifted**
**1 tbsp cocoa, sifted**
**150ml/¼pt Greek yoghurt**
**1 tbsp icing sugar, sifted**
**250g/9oz assorted berries**

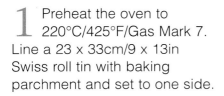

1 Preheat the oven to 220°C/425°F/Gas Mark 7. Line a 23 x 33cm/9 x 13in Swiss roll tin with baking parchment and set to one side.

2 In a large mixing bowl, whisk the eggs and sugar together until they become light and creamy in colour and the mixture leaves a "ribbon" briefly across the top when the whisk is lifted out.

3 Gently fold in the flour and cocoa with a large metal spoon. Pour the mixture into the prepared tin and bake in the preheated oven for 12–15 minutes or until it is well risen and springy to the touch.

4 Lay a large sheet of greaseproof paper on the work surface and sprinkle lightly with a little caster sugar. Turn the cooked sponge onto this and loosely roll up, discarding the lining paper as you do so. Leave to cool.

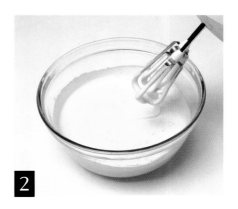

5 Beat the Greek yoghurt and icing sugar together. Unroll the roulade and spread with the sweetened yoghurt. Scatter over the berries and roll back up. Serve.

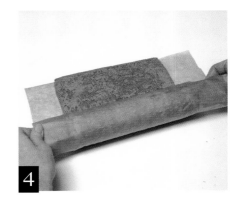

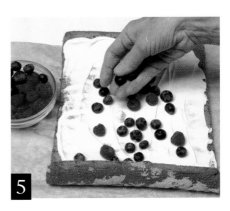

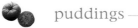 

# Baked Apples

*Low Fat*

One of these would count as one of your daily fruit and vegetable requirements.

### Serves 2

**2 large cooking apples**
**2 tbsp chopped nuts, toasted**
**2 tbsp soft brown sugar**
**25g/1oz sultanas**
**crème fraîche to serve**

### Serves 4

**4 large cooking apples**
**4 tbsp chopped nuts, toasted**
**4 tbsp soft brown sugar**
**50g/2oz sultanas**
**crème fraîche to serve**

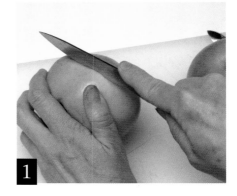

1 Preheat the oven to 180°C/350°F/Gas Mark 4. Wash and dry the apples. With a sharp knife, cut lightly through the skin about halfway up each apple, going around the circumference. Remove the core and place each apple in a piece of baking parchment that is big enough to wrap around it.

2 In a mixing bowl, blend the remaining ingredients together. Divide this mixture between the apples, spooning it in to the cavity where the core was. Sprinkle 1 tbsp of water over each apple.

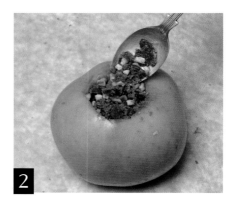

3 Bring the baking parchment up round each apple and pinch the edges together to seal. Bake in the preheated oven for 25–30 minutes. Serve piping hot, with a little crème fraîche if desired.

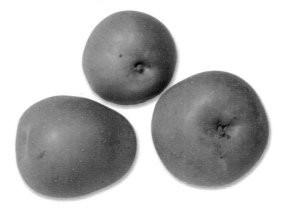

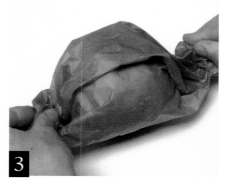

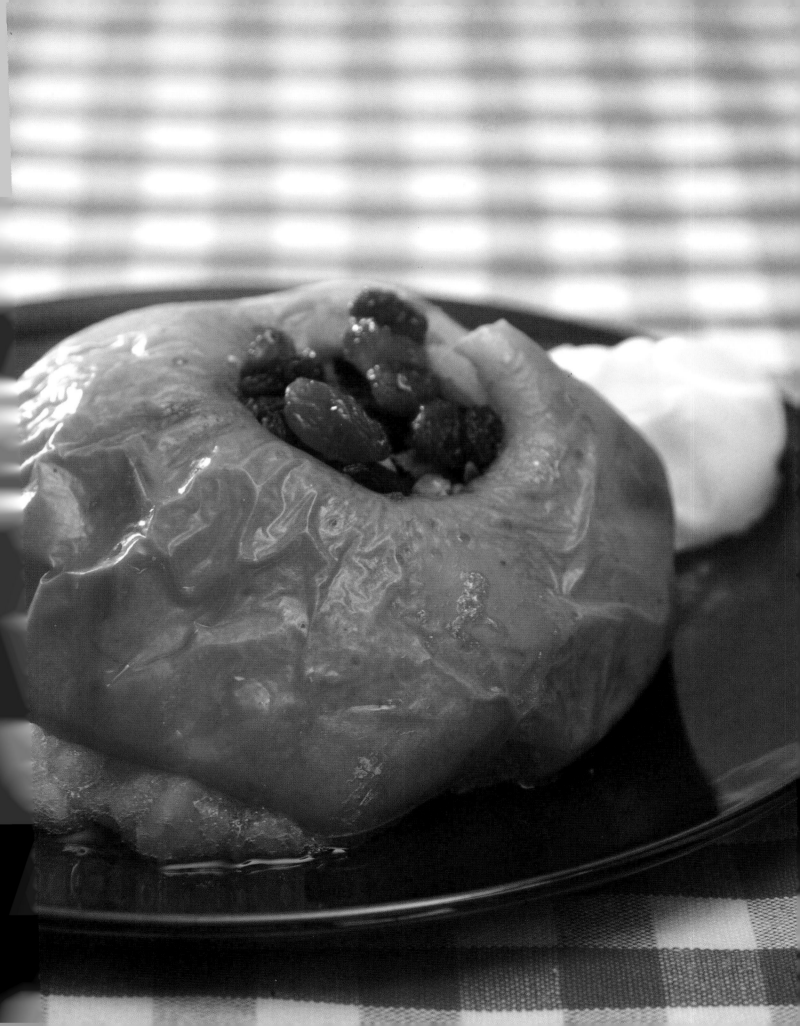

# Chocolate, Pear & Ginger Sponge

*Low Fat*

The good news is that chocolate is good for you! Not too much, obviously, but a little dark chocolate is said to help in reducing cholesterol.

## Serves 4

**100g/4oz caster sugar**
**100g/4oz butter, softened**
**100g/4oz self-raising flour**
**½ tsp baking powder**
**2 eggs, beaten**
**50g/2oz dark chocolate chunks**
**1 piece preserved stem ginger, finely chopped**
**2 large ripe pears**
**2 bananas**

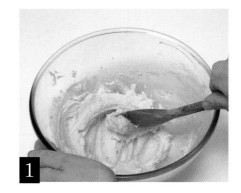

1 Preheat the oven to 180°C/350°F/Gas Mark 4. Sift the caster sugar into a mixing bowl and add the butter. Beat together with a wooden spoon until it becomes light and fluffy.

2 Sift the flour and baking powder together. Beat a little of the beaten eggs into the creamed butter and sugar and add a little of the flour and baking powder. Continue this process until all the flour and eggs have been incorporated. Fold in the chocolate and ginger.

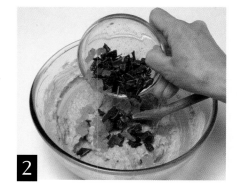

3 Peel and core the pears and peel the bananas. Chop them both into bite-size pieces. Divide the prepared fruit between four oven-proof bowls.

4 Divide the sponge mixture between the four bowls, spreading it to the edges to cover the fruit. Bake in the preheated oven for 25 minutes. Serve.

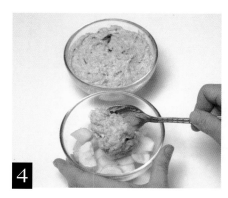

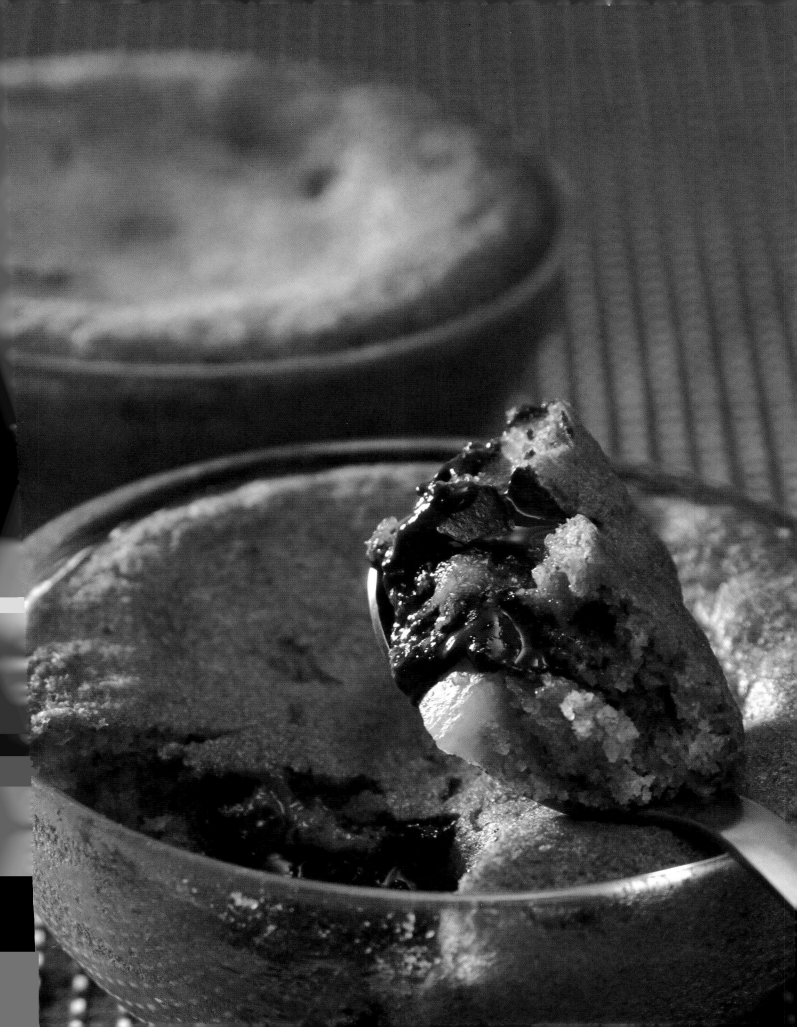

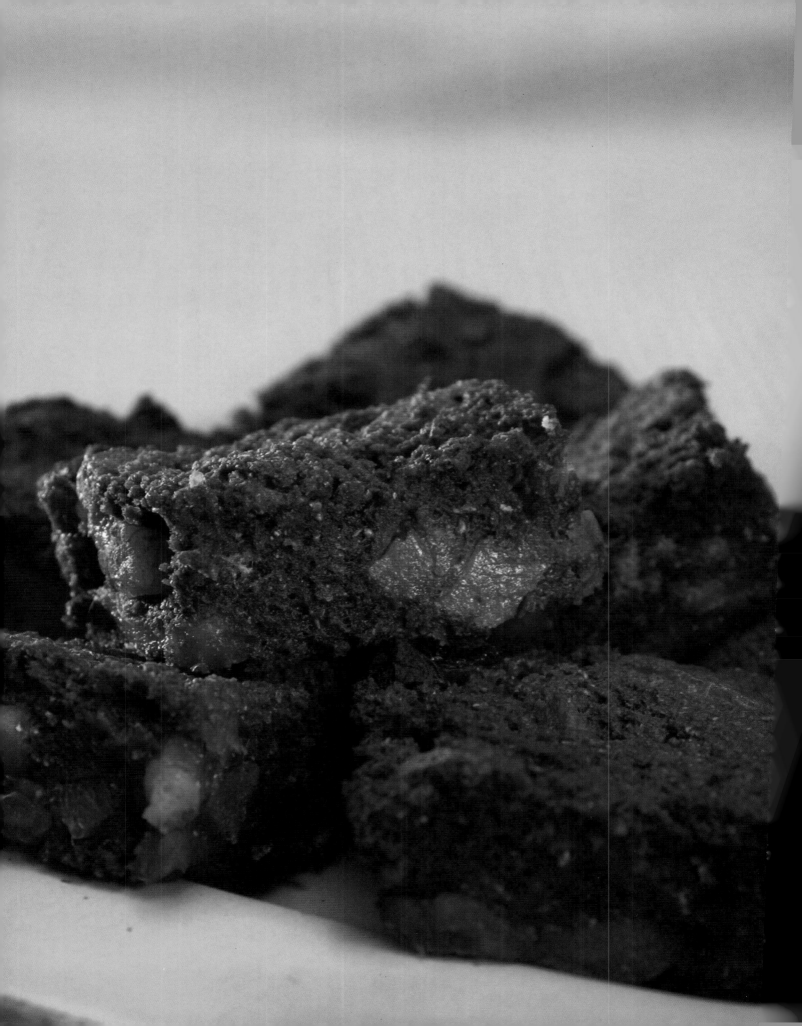

# Apricot & Mocha Bread Pudding

*Children's Choice*

This is as good cold as it is hot. Great in lunch boxes.

## Serves 6-8

**250g/9oz wholemeal bread, crusts removed**
**300ml/½pt semi-skimmed milk**
**25g/1oz cocoa**
**2 tsp espresso powder**
**75g/3oz soft dark brown sugar**
**50g/2oz butter melted**
**1 egg, beaten**
**225g/8oz dried ready-to-eat apricots, chopped**

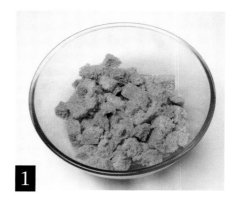

1 Roughly chop the bread and place in a large mixing bowl. Gently heat the milk until almost boiling, then remove from the heat.

2 Sift the cocoa into a small mixing bowl. Add the espresso powder and sugar, and mix. Add a little of the warmed milk and stir to form a smooth paste. Add the remaining milk, the melted butter and eggs, and mix thoroughly. Pour over the bread and set to one side for 15 minutes to soak.

3 Lightly grease a shallow baking dish. Preheat the oven to 180°C/350°F/Gas Mark 4. Stir the chopped apricots into the bread mixture and pour into the prepared baking dish. Leave to soak for a further 15 minutes.

4 Bake in the preheated oven for 1 hour. Can be served hot or cold.

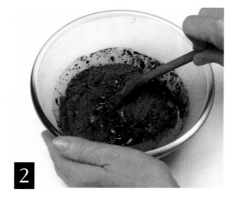

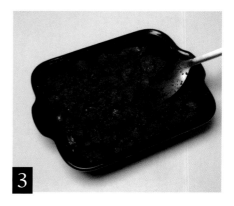

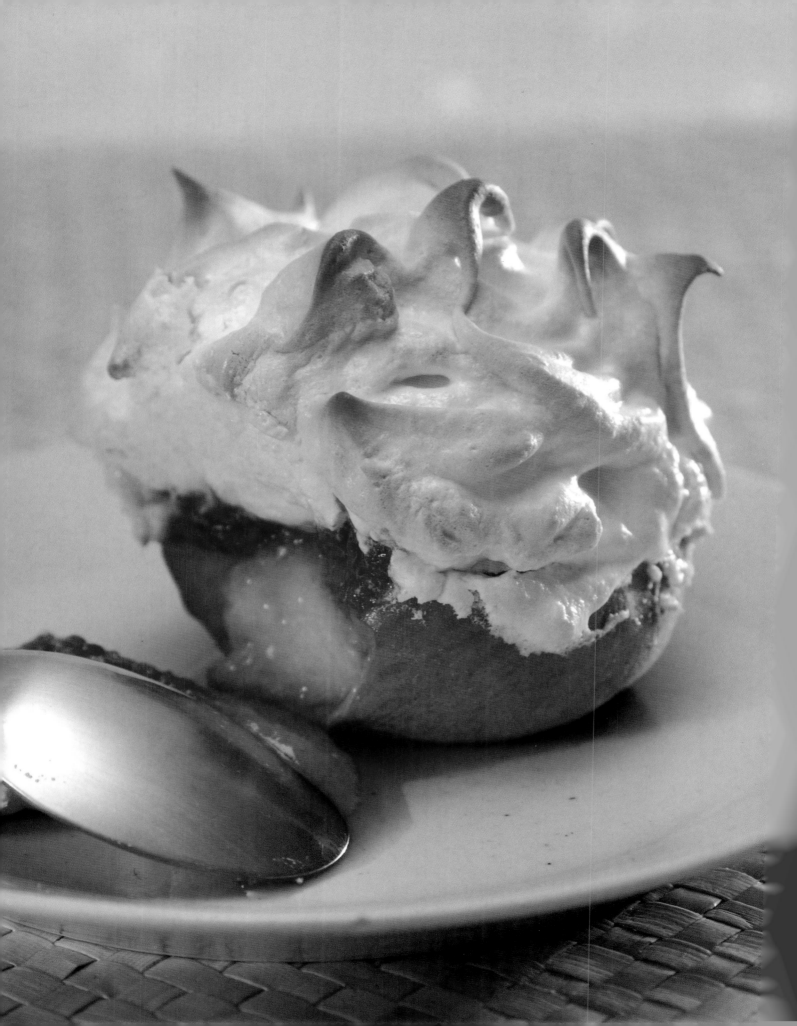

# Raspberry & Peach Meringues

*Easy Entertaining*

Peaches and raspberries go perfectly together.

### Serves 2

**1 large peach**
**50g/2oz fresh raspberries**
**½ tbsp Cointreau (optional)**
**½ egg white**
**25g/1oz caster sugar**

### Serves 4

**2 large peaches**
**100g/4oz fresh raspberries**
**1 tbsp Cointreau (optional)**
**1 egg white**
**50g/2oz caster sugar**

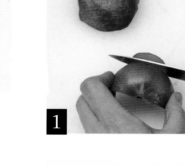

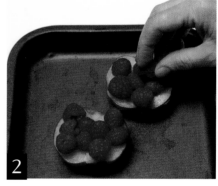

1 Preheat the oven to 190°C/375°F/Gas Mark 5. Cut the peach(es) in half and remove the stone. Place cut side up on a baking tray. If you find the peaches roll to one side, cut a thin slither from the base to help steady them.

2 Divide the raspberries between each peach half and drizzle with the Cointreau if using. Bake in the preheated oven for 15 minutes.

3 While the peaches are cooking, place the egg white in a large, grease-free mixing bowl and whisk until it forms stiff peaks. Now add the sugar 1 tbsp at a time, whisking well between each addition, until the mixture is stiff and glossy and all the sugar has been incorporated.

4 Remove the peaches from the oven and increase the oven temperature to 220°C/425°F/Gas Mark 7. Top the peaches with the meringue mixture and swirl to form little peaks. Return to the oven and cook for a further 5–7 minutes, until the meringue is golden in places. Serve.

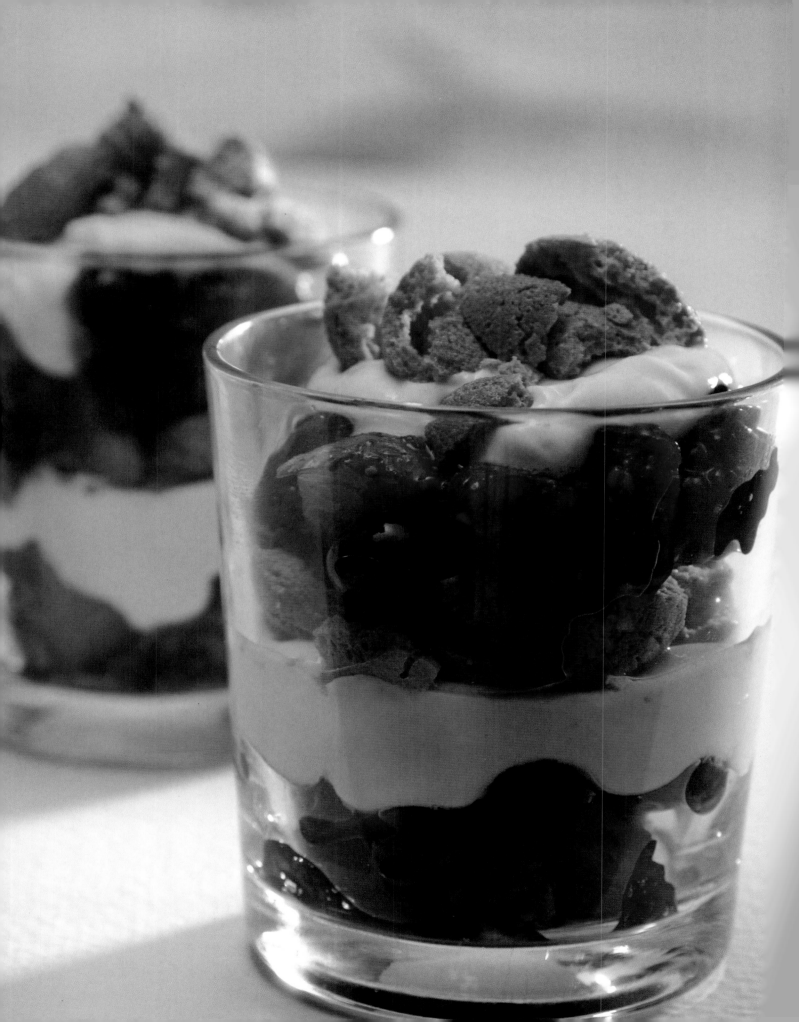

# Berry Fool

## Children's Choice

This is so easy that maybe the children could make it with just a little supervision.

### Serves 2

**225g/8oz mixed summer berries**
**150ml/¼pt Greek yoghurt**
**1 tbsp icing sugar**
**¼ tsp vanilla essence**
**6 amaretti biscuits**

### Serves 4

**450g/1lb mixed summer berries**
**300ml/½pt Greek yoghurt**
**2 tbsp icing sugar**
**½ tsp vanilla essence**
**12 amaretti biscuits**

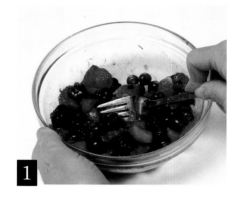

1 Roughly crush the berries with a fork. Beat the Greek yoghurt, icing sugar and vanilla essence together. Crush the amaretti biscuits and set to one side.

2 Take 2 (4) tall serving glasses and spoon a layer of the berries into the bottom of each one.

3 Top this with a thin layer of the sweetened Greek yoghurt, followed by a layer of the crushed amaretti.

4 Repeat the layers one more time, finishing with a layer of the amaretti. Serve.

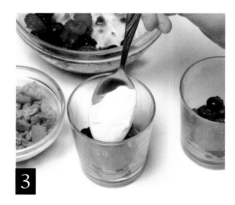

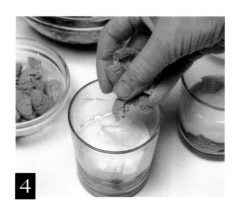

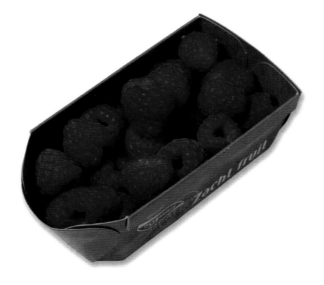

# Strawberry Sorbet

*Low Fat*

Sorbets are light and refreshing. If you can, make this when English strawberries are in season.

## Serves 4

**450g/1lb strawberries**
**90g/3½oz caster sugar**
**2 tablespoons liquid glucose**

1 Wash and hull the strawberries, then slice or roughly chop before blending to a purée in a liquidiser or food processor.

2 Place the sugar in a pan with 100ml/3½fl oz water. Heat gently, stirring, until the sugar has dissolved. Remove from the heat and set to one side to cool fully. Now combine the strawberries, syrup and liquid glucose.

3 Pour into a shallow freezer-proof container and freeze until the edges become icy. Remove from the freezer and, using a fork, stir the ice crystals through the mixture until it is all fully combined. Return it to the freezer.

4 Repeat this procedure 2–3 times. Then freeze until ready to serve. Alternatively, if you have an ice-cream maker, pour the mixture into your ice-cream maker at the end of step 2 and follow the manufacturer's instructions.

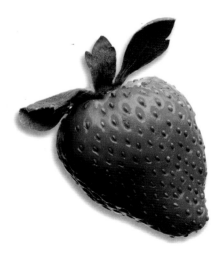

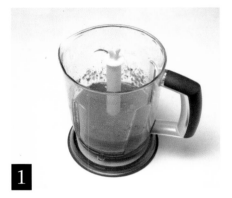

1

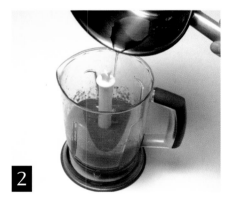

2

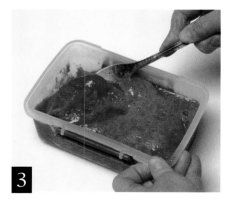

3

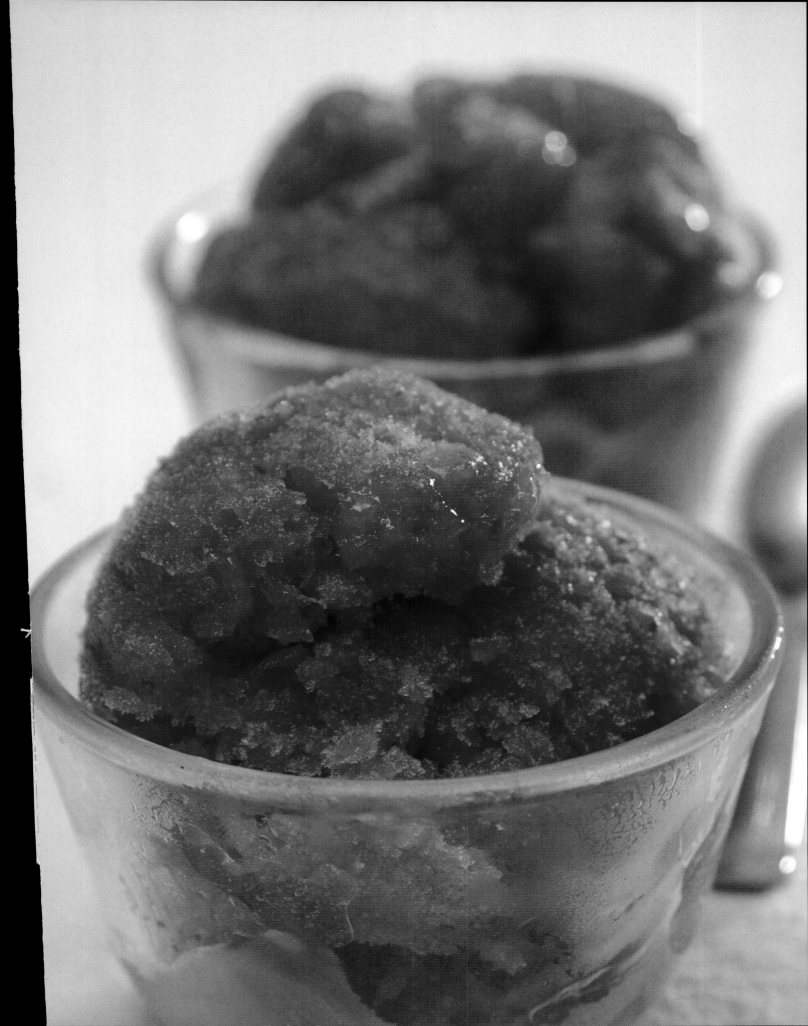

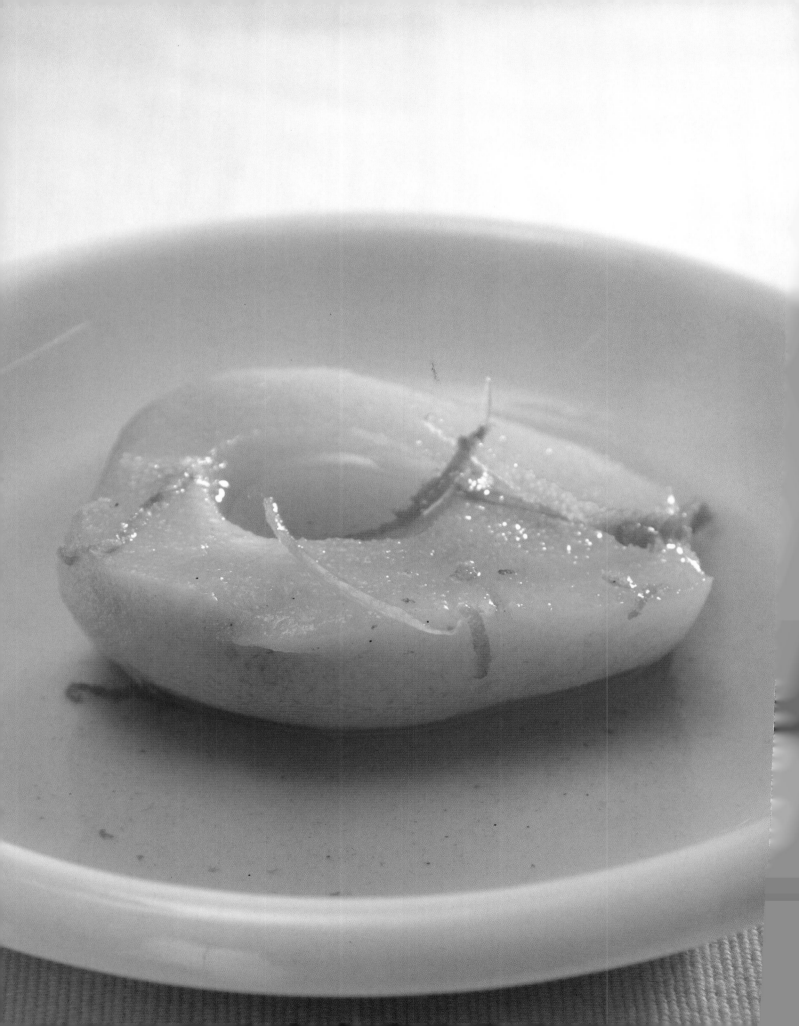

# Spiced Poached Pears

*Easy Entertaining*

This low-fat pudding is very simple to prepare.

### Serves 2

½ tbsp granulated sugar
1 star anise
½ vanilla pod, split
½ small cinnamon stick
½ orange
1 large ripe pear
crème fraîche to serve

### Serves 4

1 tbsp granulated sugar
2 star anise
1 vanilla pod, split
1 small cinnamon stick
1 orange
2 large ripe pears
crème fraîche to serve

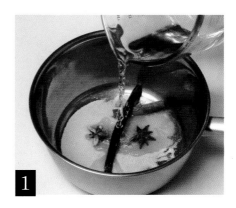

1 Place the sugar in a large saucepan with 150ml/¼pt (300ml/½pt) cold water. Add the star anise, vanilla pod and cinnamon stick.

2 Zest the orange using a zester. Alternatively, using a sharp knife, cut thin strips from the orange skin, ensuring you do not get any of the white pith. Add the zest to the pan, along with the juice from the orange.

3 Bring gently to the boil, stirring from time to time to ensure that the sugar is fully dissolved. Peel, halve and core the pears. Add to the spiced

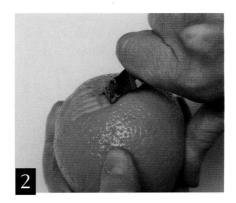

orange syrup in the pan. Cook, covered, at a gentle simmer for 20 minutes, turning the pears from time to time to ensure they are cooked through.

4 To serve, place a pear half on each plate and keep warm. Bring the cooking liquid back to a rapid boil and cook for 3–4 minutes to reduce by about half. Remove from the heat. Spoon the spiced syrup over the pears, along with a little crème fraîche.

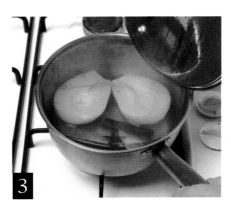

# Peach & Banana Crumble

## Children's Choice

Crumbles are one of those puddings that never fail to please.

### Serves 4

100g/4oz wholemeal self-raising flour
50g/2oz rolled oats
100g/4oz butter
75g/3oz demerara sugar
25g/1oz dessicated coconut
2 x 400g/14oz cans sliced peaches in natural juice.
2 ripe bananas

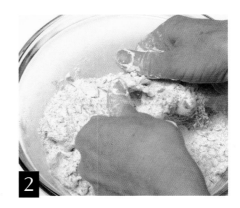

1 Preheat the oven to 200°C/400°F/Gas Mark 6. Lightly grease an ovenproof dish. Place the flour and oats together in a large mixing bowl. Cut the butter into small pieces and add to the flour and oats.

2 Lightly and quickly rub the butter into the flour until the mixture resembles coarse breadcrumbs. Stir in the sugar and dessicated coconut, then set to one side.

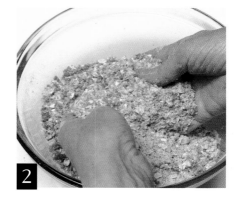

3 Drain the juice from one of the cans of peaches and discard. Pour the remaining juice into the prepared ovenproof dish along with all of the peaches. Thickly slice the bananas and scatter over the peaches.

4 Cover the fruit with the flour and oat mixture, using a fork to spread the mixture evenly. Do not press the crumble mixture down. Bake in the preheated oven for 30–35 minutes, until golden and crisp. Serve.

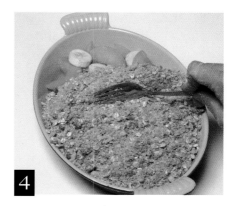

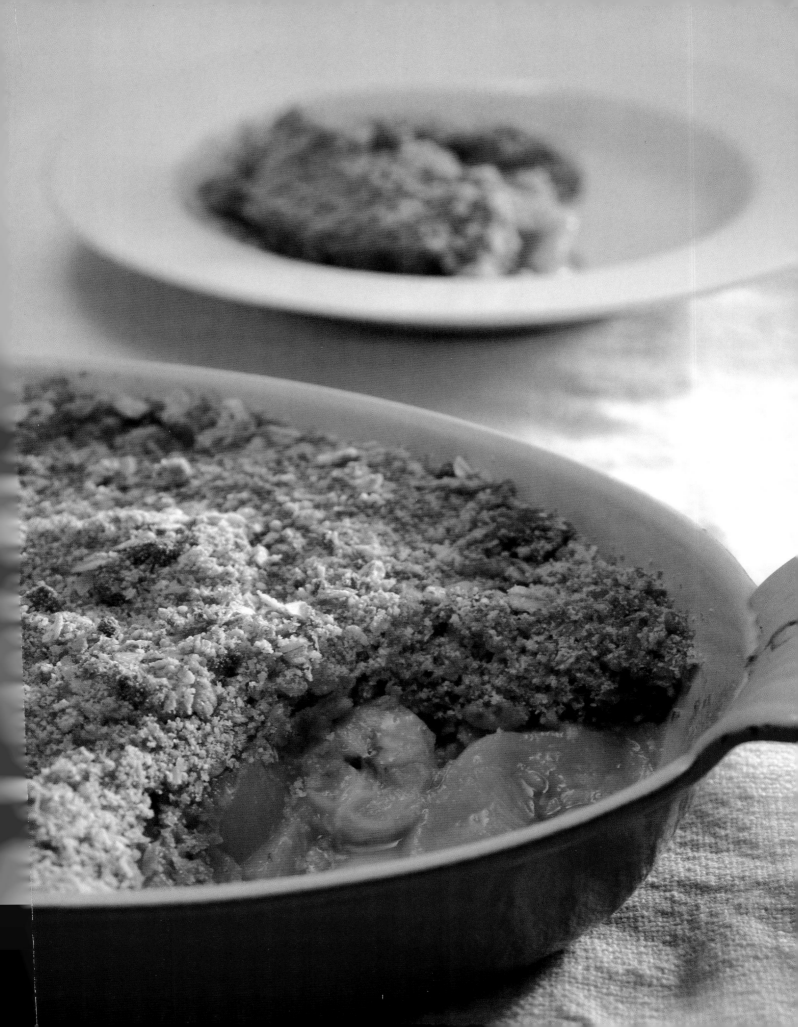

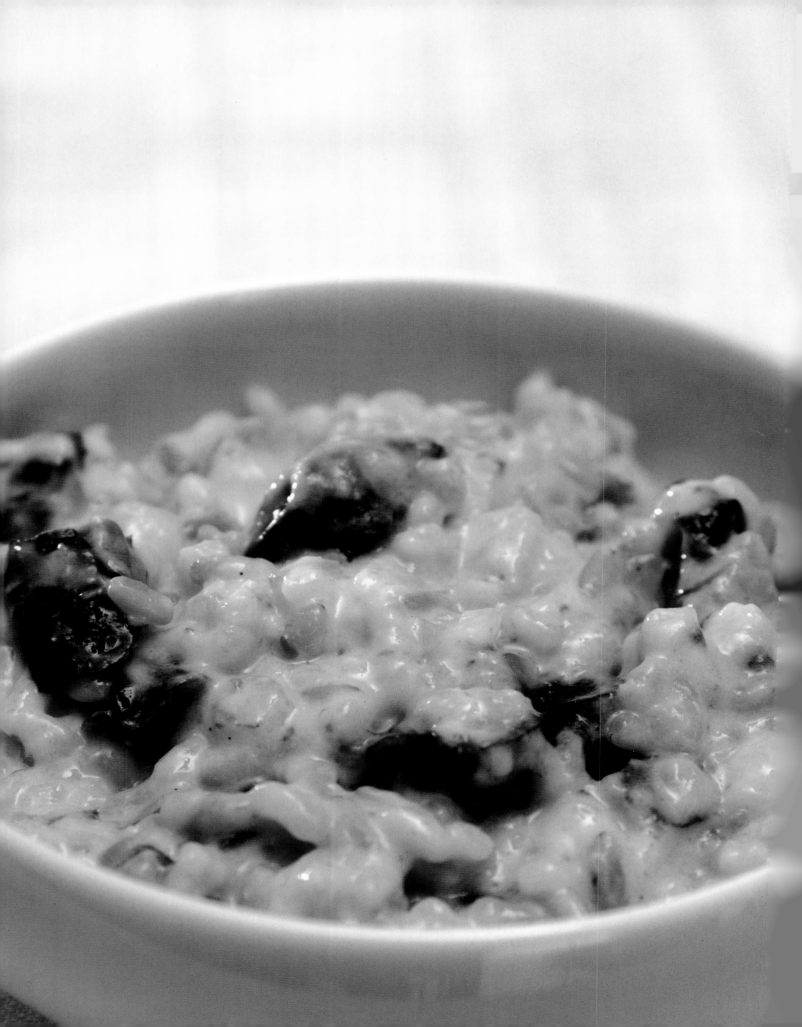

# Vanilla Rice Pudding

*One Pot*

This is delicious hot or at room temperature.

Serves 4

**1 vanilla pod**
**60g/2½oz brown rice**
**50g/2oz pudding rice**
**600ml/1pt semi-skimmed milk**
**40g/1½oz golden caster sugar**
**125g/4½oz French soft prunes, chopped**

1 Using a sharp knife, split the vanilla pod to reveal the seeds inside. Place the vanilla pod in a large saucepan with a well-fitting lid.

2 Rinse the brown rice thoroughly, then drain and add to the pan along with the pudding rice. Pour over the milk and place over a moderate heat. Bring gently to the boil, reduce the heat to a gentle simmer, cover and cook, stirring from time to time, for 40–45 minutes until the rice is tender.

3 Remove from the heat and stir in the sugar. Carefully remove the vanilla pod. Gently fold through the chopped prunes and serve hot or at room temperature.

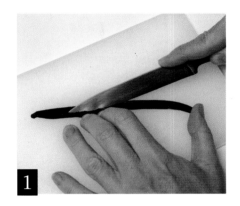

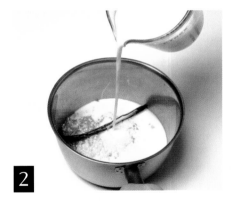

# Frozen Banana Bites

## Children's Choice

When bananas are frozen they become even more creamy in texture.

### Serves 2

**2 large ripe bananas**
**25g/1oz dark chocolate**
**15g/½oz chopped nuts**

### Serves 4

**4 large ripe bananas**
**50g/2oz dark chocolate**
**25g/1oz chopped nuts**

1 Thickly slice the bananas and place on a non-stick baking tray in the freezer for 4–6 hours or until frozen.

2 When the bananas are frozen, break the chocolate into small pieces and place in a heatproof bowl over a pan of gently simmering water, ensuring that the base of the bowl is not touching the water. Stir until the chocolate is fully melted. Remove from the heat and set to one side.

3 Place the nuts in a small frying pan and cook over a moderate heat until lightly toasted. Remove from the pan immediately to stop them from cooking further.

4 Divide the banana pieces between 2 (4) serving plates. Drizzle over the melted chocolate and sprinkle with the toasted nuts. Serve.

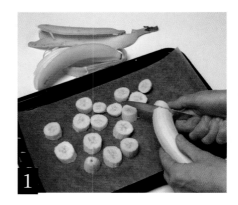

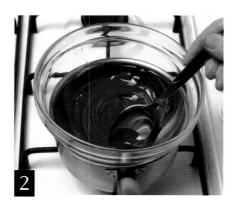

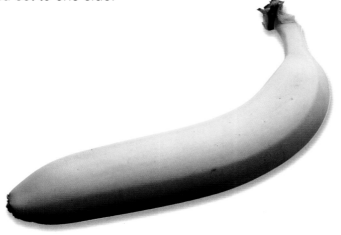

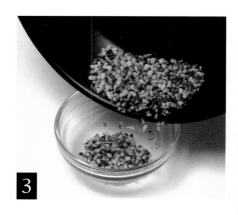

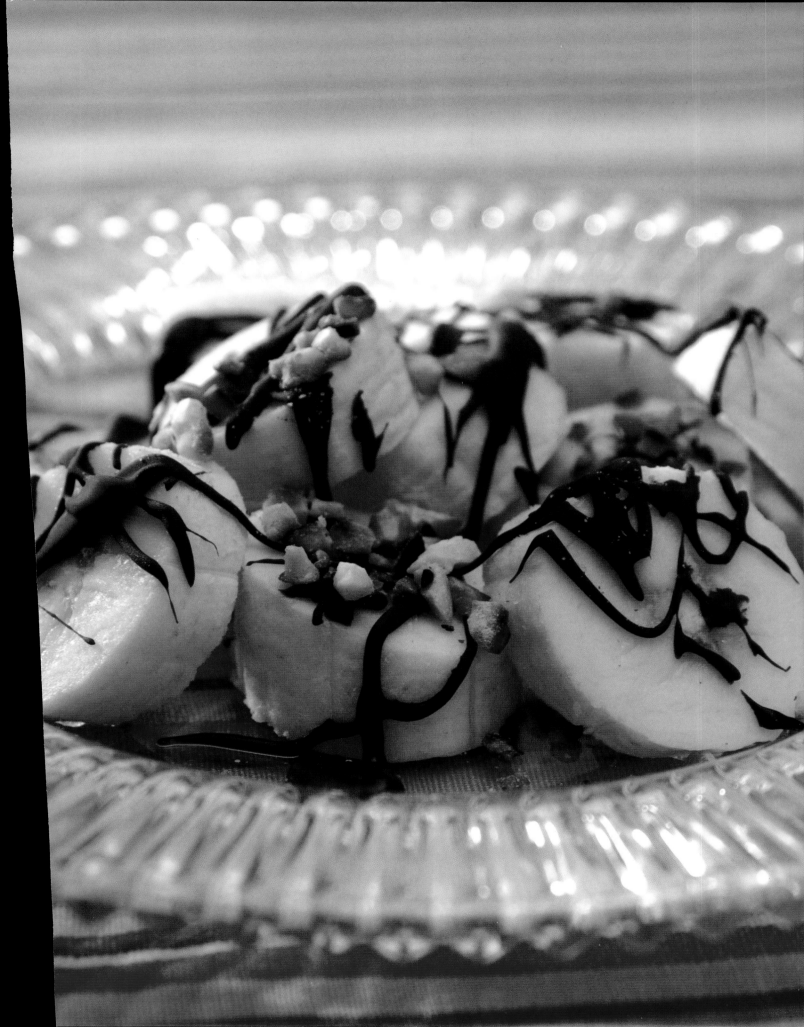

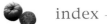
# index

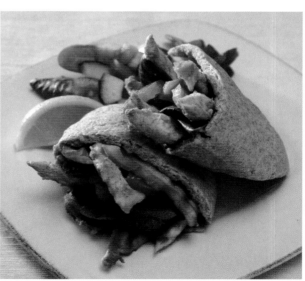

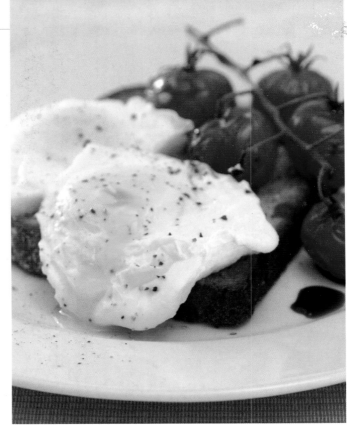

# credits & acknowledgements

Thanks to Harrison Fisher and Co (www.premiercutlery.co.uk) for supplying the knives and some of the small kitchen utensils used for the step-by-step pictures. Also thanks to Magimix whose food processor has well and truly earned its place on my kitchen worktop, making light work of the soups and some of the other dishes in this book. And thanks to Braun for the Multiquick, which was invaluable in preparing so many of the recipes.

I would also like to thank my family and Colin Bowling for all their interest, support and encouragement.